What others say

"Alzheimer's: A Beautiful [...] lovely story of discovery [...] looking at dementia, explores the pitfalls of falling into society's labels and judgments and in the end finds not only more joy in relating to her mother but also a higher level of spirituality in herself."
Vicki de Klerk-Rubin, Certified Validation Master, Validation Training Institute Board Member

"This beautiful book is about opening our minds, our hearts and our connections with others. It offers a deep exploration of the meaning of love, presence and peace amidst the challenges of dementia. Linn Possell reminds us to always continue to discover and celebrate what is possible in a relationship. This book should be shared with everyone affected by dementia."
Kelly Smith Papa, MSN, RN, Director of Education and Consulting Alzheimer's Resource Center of Connecticut

"A very readable and insightful guide to a compassionate understanding of dementia. The section on prayer is both elevating and transformative. Should be close by the side of anyone who is experiencing the decline of a loved one into the darkness of dementia."
Rev Dr Patrick J Powers, Dean, Knowles Memorial Chapel. Rollins College

"This is a soulful love story which gives practical guidance as together you enter into each other's fears and heartbreak, find personal self-forgetfulness, and the presence of the eternal within the realm of dementia. She picks areas of natural frustration for the caregiver such as the forgetfulness about our daily visits, meant to guide our new behaviors and responses thus encouraging us to step away from conflict and reinvent new ways to encounter love and protect."
Irena Delahunty, PSY. D., M.Div, STM, MA, RN Chaplain of Alzheimer's Resource Center of Connecticut

"In this ground breaking outside-the-box book, The Rev. Linn Possell shows us the way to maintain and develop a rich and rewarding relationship with loved ones with Alzheimer's. Want to know what LIFE and LOVE is? Read this book."

The Rev. Victoria N. M. Klassen, pastor, hospital chaplain, former Director of the Florida Southern College Charlotte-DeSoto Campus and Liberal Arts Bachelor Degree Program, Director of The Clearing Study Center.

"Linn has remarkable insight into the dynamics of relationships touched by this most dreaded disease. Linn's challenge to know, accept, and care for her mother as she is newly revealed through the changes in her brain, leads to a journey that brings courage and hope to those facing a similar future. I urge you to read this little book that has the power to change the lives for the better."

Fran Porter, a daughter and sister of a loved one with Alzheimer's disease.

Alzheimer's

A Beautiful Spirit Celebrated

Linn Possell

Richardson Publishing, Inc. , Altamonte Springs, Florida

Alzheimer's: A Beautiful Spirit Celebrated
Linn Possell
ISBN: 978-1-935683-23-0

Disclaimer:

Cover photograph used by permission of:
Emily Mason & Margarit Mason

Cover design / Interior layout design:
Rik Feeney
www.PublishingSuccessOnline.com

Editorial:
Maureen Jung
www.wordspringconsulting.com

Acknowledgments

I would like to say thank you to the amazing people who cared for my mother at the Alzheimer's Resource Center of Connecticut. I believe that my mother was well because she lived with this wonderful staff and because they gave her the grace and freedom to "Be". Special thanks to Elana Butler, Brittany Crane, Jennfier D'Eugenio, Donna Fielding, Sean Gavin, Nelly Jehnings, Lori MaClean, Jeannine McKenna, Taylor Parker, Christine Pilitowski, Patrycja Sudyka , and Doris Uzanas. Thanks also to Pam Atwood who worked with our family and referred us to the center.

Thank you to Judy Peterson and Terry Wolfe who helped me through the initial stage of my mother's illness. And to my family... we were given the gift of a beautiful spirit.

To my friends and family who supported and encouraged me to write this book because they believed I had something to share that could help others affected by Alzheimer's and dementia...thank you; Stephanie Possell, Lois Hasty, Randi Solomon, Barbara Antidormi, Denise Clark, Maudi Sauza and Victoria Klassen.

Dedication

For my mother Elaine, and my partner Stephanie.

Table of Contents

FOREWORD

Here is the story of one person's experience with Alzheimer's. Not all people who have Alzheimer's experience the same issues that the author or her mother did; nor do all people with frontal-temporal dementia share them. I'd wager everyone in the author's family experienced things differently. Because of our own unique human development, each of us experiences diseases like Alzheimer's uniquely. The danger of books about personal accounts is they do not always provide a perspective that is universally shared. Yet, I am reflecting on a support group meeting from earlier this week. As the group's facilitator, I was thinking of our members: some members care for a parent, some for a spouse, and others for siblings; some care for people at the end of life, others at the beginning of the disease process. Each would benefit from reading this book. One woman was there for the first time – reaching out after confessing to her best friend about her mother's changes. In her very lonely time, she especially would benefit from reading this book.

The crisis of Alzheimer's and other forms of dementia is truly a crisis of spirit. It is a challenge to our personhood, our tolerance, often our physical strength as well as our strength of character. Ultimately it challenges our own ego integrity when we question, "Am I the kind of person who can handle the challenge to *celebrate* the spirit of someone who changes?" As Rev Possell alludes to, the reason Alzheimer's is "hard" is not simply because we slowly watch someone we love struggle with change and loss, but that Alzheimer's also requires US to change. Obviously, the person with the dementia changes, and intellectually we understand that is inevitable; for those changes and losses we grieve. The real challenge comes in our ability to change ourselves for the person who struggles with the disease. Can we change: our expectations, our relationships, our comfort, sometimes our definition of security or "home" and finally, our ability to celebrate a spirit less familiar? The disease challenges us to see beyond the person we know, accept their vulnerabilities and to hold them sacred.

In reading this book, quite beautifully the author creates ways for readers to reflect. She provides opportunities to explore connection with our loved ones. In sharing her personal and singular experience, we all relate and reflect. Even if our experience is not matched issue by issue, the opportunities to celebrate a spirit are illuminated by comparison to her journey.

In our support group, we often talk about the evolution of ourselves as caregivers. The wisdom Rev Possell shares enables readers to rapidly evolve to become effective caregivers. As a reader, you will learn to be angry at a disease, not a person. You will feel compelled to advocate for loved ones instead of accepting labels and stereotypes. You realize the challenges are internal as well as in a moment. Most importantly, you will learn that celebration of a spirit is the joy of quietly considering a soul on a level much deeper than occupation, learned skills or fluency. It's celebrating through listening, reaching, needing, and in being with, and for another. The true celebration of that spirit is how a person, so deeply affected by a horrifying disease, can still teach us to be better human beings.

~ **Pamela Krist Atwood**, MA, Certified Dementia Practitioner, Suppport Group leader, and former caregiver, Director of Dementia Care Services, Hebrew Health Care, West Hartford, CT.

INTRODUCTION

Our Spirit continues toward growth and awareness

"Open my eyes that I may see, glimpses of truth thou hast for me. Open my eyes illumine me, Spirit Divine." Clara H. Scott

My mother is the kind of teacher who was born to teach. She embodies everything that makes a teacher great. She is patient and flexible, which gives her the ability to adapt her teaching to the kind of instruction that students need. My mother is committed and demanding and holds her students to the highest standards. She is accepting of and celebrates diversity and has been recognized for her work with the curriculum "Teaching Tolerance." She instructs from her knowledge and teaches from her heart. My mother has always been one of my greatest teachers, whether she was instructing me how to write an essay or teaching me about life. Therefore it is no surprise to me that, after my mother's diagnosis of frontal-lobe dementia in 2006, I have continued to learn my most valuable lessons from her. What I learn from her now is about the expression of our soul and our capacity for spiritual connectedness.

I have learned that how we understand and recognize the expression of our soul and the extent to which we are able to connect spiritually with another's life stems from our openness to this experience. My hope is to help others embrace a different way of experiencing and interacting with their loved ones who have dementia or Alzheimer's disease and to trust in the possibility of staying spiritually connected to them throughout their time with us. Regardless of cognitive decline, our soul continues to find expression and our spiritual essence continues toward growth and awareness. Even in the midst of this disease, we can find a beautiful connection with one another.

Alzheimer's and dementia are usually considered barriers that keep us from connecting with our loved one and leave us feeling as if they do not know how much we love them. When a family member is diagnosed with dementia or Alzheimer's, the family may feel as if they are being left behind. They may fear that they will not be able to have a meaningful relationship with their mother, father, spouse or sibling. But it is possible to have a beautiful relationship with our loved one even when they have this disease, if we can look for and find ways that foster this connection. If it is our goal to continue to relate to and connect with our loved one, we must be open to change. A meaningful relationship will happen when we are open to changing our perception about this disease and open to finding new ways for connection to take place.

It is my hope that this book will help families affected by cognitive impairment celebrate and embrace the life of their loved one. Dementia has been called "the long goodbye" because it takes away pieces that make up the identity of an individual. It also creates a sense of helplessness as we, the families, watch what we know as the identity of our loved one and their ways of relating to us appear to fade away. I continue to see family members who grieve on a daily basis. They grieve because to them, their loved one has died. However, I believe that "the long goodbye" distracts us from living life in the present moment. I personally feel that the phrase "the long goodbye" has the potential to disvalue the life of the person with the disease. It is, in a sense, a way of saying that if someone cannot continue to live the way they once did, that their life is somehow diminished. Dementia *does* change the way a person lives, but it does not take away the *value* of a life.

With Alzheimer's and dementia come many struggles. One struggle is that they slowly take away many of a person's abilities and functions. This is difficult for both the person who has the disease and their family and loved ones. It was very difficult for my mother when she began to lose her language, because she knew that she was not able to retrieve her words. Communication, which was always effortless for my mother, now required a great deal of effort. I remember how painful it was for me to watch her struggle to find words. Seeing a loved one struggle while knowing that we are, for the most part, helpless in fixing the problem is hard for many of us. One of the lessons that I have learned as my mother's disease progressed is how to deal with something that doesn't have any perfect answers. As family members, we need to be patient with ourselves and with our loved one, and instead of becoming frustrated, focus on we can do for both of us.

At some point, losses become more painful for the family members than for the person with the disease. It is important to observe our loved one and recognize when they are no longer affected by their losses, so that we do not transfer our pain to them. Furthermore, if we can rethink how we perceive these changes and decline, then we may be able to heal the pain that accompanies this disease.

Some of the most difficult things for family members and loved ones to experience are the person's inability to retrieve memory, the loss of recognition, and the perceived lack of emotion. These changes are difficult because they are verbal and nonverbal cues that we have always used to help us feel connected and to help us know that we are important to one another. Relationships and connecting with another person feel more difficult without these cues. Therefore, it is my goal to help families go beyond our familiar ways of connecting to our loved one and find new ways to know that we are significant in one another's life. Even though our relationship will look different and the ways in which we relate to one another will change, our relationship will be rich and meaningful as we learn how to open our eyes to the soul and reach out to touch the spirit.

A CHANGE IN PERCEPTION

Looking Beyond

"We pass by the joys of life without knowing we've missed anything." Yang Chu

Joy of life comes from being open to finding ways of connecting with one another and by expressing our love for each other. My life has changed because of my personal experience of learning how to engage, connect with, and celebrate the life of my mother who has Frontotemporal dementia. I always had a very close relationship with my mother, because we were similar in almost every way. The fact that we were so similar was, for me, a source of security in who I was as a person, because I thought that my mother was capable of doing anything and because everyone loved her. I felt that if I was anything at all like my mother, I would be okay. Our similarities also caused us both a lot of frustration, which is very common for mothers and daughters who are a lot alike. I believe that our relationship and our similarities have helped me observe and in some ways understand her experience.

When I realized that my mother was losing her ability to interact with me in traditional and familiar ways, I knew that it was up to me to learn what she was able to understand and how best to relate to her. My number one priority was to let my mom know that I loved her and to finds ways that would help her feel that no matter what happened, she would be okay. I remember being out by my pool with my mother one day when she could not find a word that she wanted to say. I remember telling her that it would be okay and that I would make it my job to find the words that she wanted to say. I told her that we would always be able to communicate with each other because I would make it my responsibility to find ways for us to do so. Saying this was both comforting to her and to me, because I was assuring my mother that I would always be there to help her, and I was assuring myself that I would be able to help with something even though I couldn't affect the disease.

Usually we connect to one another through a variety of social interactions, by sharing a history together, and through common interests. But what happens when we are no longer able to use these common avenues? Can we go beyond these and find other points of connection? If we want to stay connected with our loved one who has dementia, it is necessary to explore other means to do so. For example, when the ability to speak is lost, we can find ways to communicate without language and without the expectation of a verbal exchange. If our loved one continues to be able to speak, but loses memory and forgets that we share a common history; we look for other things to share.

Awareness and understanding can help limit the amount of frustration we feel when we interact with a person who has dementia. This disease can cause our loved one to begin to lose interest in things that once were important to them. It can even seem as if they lack interest in most everything. Understanding that this is part of the disease can help us realize that when we see a lack of interest in a hobby or activity, for example, we need to look for a different activity that they find interesting or to which they will respond. An old interest or activity can change from a way to connect and engage with our mother, father, sibling or spouse, to being a source of frustration. If this happens, we can substitute a new interest and experiment with things to which they might respond.

One Mother's Day, when my mother was still able to live at home, I took her to buy flowers for her front yard. My mother always loved to plant flowers and we would often go together to get flowers to plant in her yard. Mother's Day that year was different. Mom was very happy to go with me and pick out flowers, but when we came home she did not want to participate in planting the flowers. Even though I tried to encourage her to be part of the activity, my mother stood watching me as I planted the flowers alone. She only wanted to hold the yard bag for me as I put some yard trash into it. It struck me as odd that mom did not want to do something that had always brought her a lot of joy. People with dementia and Alzheimer's will withdraw from activities for several reasons. What is important for us as loved ones is to realize when they need, and when they will accept, gentle reminders about how to be engaged in an activity. It is also important to know when to allow them to be comfortable as observers. My mother was still part of the activity of planting the flowers as an observer, and she seemed to be okay with that. One thing that we can do is to follow their lead while also keeping options open, because their level of being engaged and interested in an activity can change from day to day.

We can also help our loved one when we give them cues about an activity. This can help them understand an activity and know what they can do to participate. For example, I began to use sign language with my mother, and that has really helped her understand and continue to be able to respond to me. I used sign language before she lost all verbal communication in hope that she might retain some of the sign language, and it seems as if that has been the case. When we were planting the flowers, for example, I opened the trash bag and gave it to her, demonstrating how she could keep it open. Our loved ones will forget how to do very simple tasks such as holding a trash bag open and therefore, if we observe a hesitation with a task, we can gently remind them how to do it.

Using sign language along with our words can also help. I used the sign language for "I love you" and "You are beautiful" with my mother as the disease progressed. Even now, in her advanced stage of the disease, she will smile when I sign to her that I love her and that she is beautiful.

Perceptions

There are thousands of individuals who live with cognitive impairment and many of them suffer in silence. An estimated 5.3 million people live with Alzheimer's disease in the US. People who have not been affected by this disease in general do not know how to communicate with or empathize with persons who have cognitive impairment and their care givers. I am often reminded of the struggle I personally had when I brought my mother into a public place where I received distressed and or frustrated looks from people who thought that her behavior was unacceptable for one reason or another. Often when we approached the entrance or walked in the door to a restaurant, people would turn and stare at my family. We were used to people staring at my mother because she was so beautiful. Now they were staring because she was what society would label "different." I used to think to myself that if they only knew her beautiful spirit, they might be more compassionate. It was sad for me to see people unaware of my "beautiful" mom, and I felt that it was my responsibility to protect her from them.

We all behave this way toward one another at times. When we are seen or we see someone else, perhaps for the first time, we immediately begin our assessment. We think: short, tall, young, old, overweight, underweight, attractive, successful, etc. We put one another into boxes and make judgments. It is very difficult for a person to live in a box; it also diminishes the life of that person.

How we identify one another

What is eternal about our life is our energy, and this energy is our spirit and our soul. In order for us to relate to one another in this human life, we place identifying markers around this energy. For example, my mother is identified by her children, her physical appearance, her role as mother, the way she speaks, her mannerisms, her occupation as a teacher, etc. We put all of these markers around her energy so that we can point to that energy and say "mom." But these markers become impediments when they become markers of loss rather than life. In order to help ourselves and our loved one affected by dementia, we need to look beyond the boxes and labels and traditional identifying markers that we have. A new possibility for life emerges as we begin to see the spirit in each other with our hearts and recognize one another in new and creative ways.

Judgments

"Out beyond the idea of wrongdoing and rightdoing there is a field. I will meet you there."
Rumi

Beyond Judgments

When we judge ourselves or another person, we stop our spiritual and emotional growth. The culture we live in is driven by this kind of judgment and the result is that both our culture and the people who live in it suffer. People suffer because the labels placed on them make their lives one dimensional.

Often times when a person has been diagnosed with a disease, the people around them begin to see them as their disease. For this reason I hesitated to name my mother's disease. I hesitated because I did not want my mother to become her disease.

Recently my mother fell and had to go to the Emergency Room. My mother walks most of the day where she lives and because her balance is somewhat impaired, she has fallen on more than one occasion. However, as a family, we have decided that we want her to continue to be able to walk for as long as possible because she finds great joy in walking throughout her day.

One night, while I was at my sister's house, we received a call telling us that mom had fallen and needed to be transported to the local hospital for a possible head injury. After I requested that my mother not be transported until we arrived, we jumped into my car and drove the 45 minutes it took to get to the hospital. Of course Connecticut was getting the first snow storm of the winter that night and the roads were slippery. But I drove as quickly as I could regardless of the snow because we did not want my mother going to the ER alone. Since my mother does not understand everything that is said to her, we did not want her to be frightened and confused being by herself in the hospital. Another difficulty is that she is fully ambulatory and puts inedible objects into her mouth. Therefore, it is not safe for my mother to be anywhere by herself. My sister and I knew that she could walk out of the ER if not watched. Driving as quickly as we could through the snow, past several accidents on the highway, we managed to get to my mother before too long. The nurse from her unit called while we were driving to tell us that because of her injuries she needed to be transported to the ER before we could arrive but they sent a Certified Nurse's Assistant to be with her much to our relief.

We found my mother sitting in a bed, with her CNA by her side, bleeding from her chin and obviously concerned about what was happening but we also received a great smile from her when we entered the room. Even with a broken nose, laceration on her chin and a broken hand, she smiled and reached for our hands. We were very relieved to see her calm and okay and were deeply touched by her ability to focus on the fact that we were there to take care of her.

I am an athletic trainer and have had similar experiences with my athletes. When an athlete goes down on the field or court with a serious injury, they will often relax when they see me coming out because they know that I will take care of them. My mother had the same reaction in the ER. She reached out to take our hands while looking at us intently, but became calmer as we smiled and told her that she was okay.

When the doctor arrived, our experience changed. He immediately asked what was wrong with my mother. The question was not about how she fell. The question was not asked regarding the gash on her chin that was bleeding profusely, nor her swollen nose. The doctor wanted to know what was "wrong" with her meaning why was she was not communicating and why she was moving her jaw back and forth. The doctor wanted to know what was "wrong" with her as if there were something "wrong" or "broken" about my mother. He did not seem to notice her injuries, and did not do a physical assessment. In fact, we had to point out my mother's hand and ask if he thought it was broken. The Doctor's focus was her dementia and his statements and actions let us know that he was not happy about having to care for her.

As my sister, mother and I waited four hours to get treatment, we were told by the ER doctor, the x-ray techs and one of the nurses that they would not be able to give her the care she needed. This included a CT, X-ray and stitches for her chin. The minute they knew she had dementia, my mother was treated as if she were a burden. The staff wanted to sedate her but never thought to give her any pain medication. My sister and I had to advocate for her and for the care she was given. The minute they began to talk about giving her sedation, I pulled out the list of medications that my mother was taking and insisted that they only give her what was approved by her doctors. I also asked them to try and care for her without extra sedation but did ask for pain medication which they seemed to have forgotten to consider. I convinced them that my mother would be able to get x-rays if I went into the room with her. Much to the tech's surprise, my mother was fine getting x-rays without being sedated.

Our ER visit was a difficult one. My sister and I watched the doctor sit outside our room for hours with no other patients to care for but my mother. My mother sat in the bed for four hours with a folded sheet on her chest to catch the blood dripping from her chin. She waited four hours to receive three stitches, three hours for pain medication and my sister and I had to try and stop the bleeding from her chin ourselves.

The frustrated and disapproving looks from people in public places and the lack of care that she received from the ER staff occurred because people did not understand her disease. They lacked awareness of, and did not seem to care to see her beautiful life. Rather than seeing my mother, they saw a woman with a disease and focused on who they thought someone with dementia and Alzheimer's is. They labeled my mother and reacted to the label and to the behaviors they expected would accompany this disease. They did not see a life of a mother who is loved and cherished, and a spirit that is celebrated by her family.

Beyond behaviors

There are some challenging and unpredictable behaviors that are manifested by dementia. These can cause a great deal of stress to families. Sometimes the behaviors seem inappropriate and cause anxiety, frustration and embarrassment. Learning about these changes in behavior can help decrease anxiety and understand that these behaviors are part of the disease, not the individual. It is helpful if we can separate the behavior from the identity of our loved one and also remember that their disease is no reflection on who we are.

Behavior changes can also be a way of signaling shifts in the progression of the disease and overall well-being. There is a lot written about behavioral changes in dementia that help us understand what the behavior is telling us. You can also learn how to respond to these changes and how to minimize the stress these changes can bring to everyone involved. This information can keep us from focusing on a troubling behavior to seeing it as a sign of something that needs to be addressed. Much of the anxiety and embarrassment that people experience when a family member exhibits dementia related behaviors comes from society.

In society, we label behaviors as acceptable or unacceptable, good or bad, as part of the system of judgment in which we live. This system of judgment is made up of societal norms, religious dogma and man-made morality. We label, judge, reward, punish, honor, and hate based on this system. While some people will argue that this system is necessary for communal life, I believe that this system fails us on many levels. It distorts life, subjugates people to the margins of life and society and reinforces the dualistic thinking that makes some people good and others bad. This system fails especially when dealing with dementia. The reason for this failure is that behaviors do not make up the essence of our being. The essence of our being is our spirit and soul, the essence of our being is life.

Behavior is usually driven by our core belief about ourselves and of the world. For example, if we believe that the world is an unfriendly place and life is something to be feared, then we live our lives based on fear. If, however, we believe that the universe moves all things toward harmony and balance and that all life is connected, then we will live a very different life. For people who have dementia the disease usually dictates the behavior and how someone lives. For instance, when a person has a brain disorder, they often use profanity but this is a sign of the disease and we must not associate the language with the person. Furthermore, people with cognitive impairment do not understand that going over to someone else's food and taking it for themselves is not acceptable or that dumping their drink on the floor is not the most helpful thing to do.

When we see an adult put an object into their mouth, we could get frustrated with that person because we think they should know better than to eat something that is inedible. If we understand these behaviors as a sign of the disease, we are better able to move to a place of compassion rather than frustration and judgment. Trying to eat an inedible object is simply a sign of dementia and does not in any way make up the essence of a person's life.

When we can change the way we see and think about a behavior and understand it as a sign of the disease rather than as an indication of a person's worth or acceptability, then we may be able to embrace what holds life together, the joys and pleasures of relationships. It is difficult to experience joy with a person who has dementia if we equate the person with the disease. But it is very possible to experience relationship when we stop judging one another. I learned this lesson one evening when I took my mother to a restaurant.

For several months my mother went through a period of wanting to put pepper on all her food. Therefore, when we went to dinner one night, I was not surprised to see her reach for the pepper mill on the table. In most restaurants we visited with my mother, there were pepper shakers so the pepper mill was more complex than she was used to. My mother reached out and took the pepper mill on the table and indicated that she wanted to put pepper on her food. However, she was unable to figure out how to get the peppermill to work. It was very difficult for some of the people at the table to watch this once capable woman confused about how to use the mill. Realizing that I could either become upset and frustrated at her obvious decline, or use this as an opportunity to engage my mother, I choose the latter.

I wanted to help my mother understand that she was still "okay" by helping her master this task. I took the pepper mill and demonstrated how to use it, then gave it back to her and let her try to work it. Because she was beginning to have difficulty understanding language, I also tried to use a minimal amount of words when helping her. This situation reminded me of trying to help my classes of middle school students learn how to tie a square knot..."right over left, no...over, over...right over left, etc." In both cases, mastery of the task required that the other person be able to complete the task alone. It would not have helped for me to tie the knot or work the pepper mill. Suffice it to say that this process took a very long time, and I had to ignore those around us as their frustration level rose with each attempt. In the end, my mother was able to use the pepper mill on her own, and I will never forget the look of joy she had when she was successful. This was a very important accomplishment for my mother, because she was able to experience being able to complete a task that had become difficult for her. It was also important for me, because I learned how much we can give to one another when we accept them as whole. For example, I could have taken the pepper mill from her and put the pepper on her meal, so we could all "get on" with our dinner but that would have sent the message that she was both unworthy of my time and incapable of performing a simple task. The messages we give to one another can have a huge impact on their quality of life.

Sum of Accomplishments

"When you reach the end of what you should know, you will be at the beginning of what you should sense." Kahlil Gibran

Our culture tells us that we are the sum of our accomplishments. Sadly, when we no longer meet the expectations of who we are, because we can no longer accomplish the same things we once did, we lose our place in society. I had a friend tell me that she felt as if she lost respect from people once she retired from her position as a computer analyst. One of the first things we do when meeting a new person is ask what they do. Knowing their profession or where they work becomes part of the identity that we give to one another. Roles are important aspects of identity in our culture. But our roles are not important aspects of our essence. My mother can no longer fulfill the "role" of mothering her children, but this in no way diminishes who she is and her importance in our life. I sometimes wonder if it would be better for us to call her by her first name rather than "mom," simply because with dementia, the memory that remains is usually the memory of our youth, and I wonder if "mom" might confuse her. In the earlier stages of her disease, she used to tell me stories of her High School days over and over again. One time she saw a picture of my brother and me, and thought that it was a picture of her and her brother.

When we believe that our accomplishments define who we are, we can lose our sense of self and our identity.

People experience all kinds of loss with Alzheimer's and the prospect of having this disease carries with it many fears: the fear of losing control, losing abilities, losing awareness, memory, connection, and ultimately losing life. But the fear of losing life is sometimes not the fear of death because many of the people with whom I have spoken in the early stage of this disease would rather die before the disease progresses. The fear of losing life is often the fear of losing the life that we know. This is one of the reasons I am writing this book.

I am very proud of my mother and her accomplishments. I have now learned there is more to celebrate, which goes beyond what we have accomplished in life. Now that I am able to see my mother beyond her accomplishments, skills and abilities, I have been able to witness the spirit that was the source of everything that she did.

I believe that who we are is about how we live, connect with others, and how we celebrate our life. I do not believe that who we are is defined by what we do. But we live in a world and culture that tell us otherwise. We are taught that life consists of what we do and our identity is determined and measured by skill, ability, and accomplishments. If our identity has always been attached to and built on our ability to do our job, for example, then when we no longer have that job... just who are we? Dementia becomes a disease that has the potential to rob us of our worth as a person, our identity and our life, and for this reason alone people fear this disease.

Getting help can be scary

I remember how difficult it was to convince my mother it was in her best interest that we take her to Mayo Clinic in an attempt to get some answers to the changes my siblings and I saw in her. When my sister and I sat down with my mother to talk with her about going to the doctor, she refused to admit that there was anything going on. She denied she was having any difficulties whatsoever. In the beginning of this disease, the signs and symptoms may be intermittent and many people cope fairly well. The signs may also look like signs of some other age related decline. There are also many reasons people are apprehensive about admitting they have signs and symptoms that might be pointing to dementia. One reason for this fear is that society places a stigma of being "less than" on individuals who experience cognitive decline.

As family members, we can be sensitive to the stigma placed on individuals with this disease. No one wants to be considered "less than." And no one *would* be considered "less than" if we were not conditioned to identify the value and worth of life by our accomplishments. Oriah Mountain Dreamer writes in her book, *The Invitation*:

> *It doesn't interest me what you do for a living. I want to know what you ache for, and if you dare to dream of meeting your heart's longing. It doesn't interest me how old you are. I want to know if you will risk looking a fool for love, for your dream, for the adventure of being alive...*

Long after the accomplishments of life have faded into the background and our loved one's ability to connect in traditional ways have gone, their life continues to be a life of beauty. Therefore, I believe that we, as the family, have a sacred responsibility to our loved one, which is to hold their life in our hearts. We are the ones who remember what their dreams and adventures were. These memories create a bond between us that enable us to find new ways of connecting that moves from one heart to another.

CHALLENGES WE ALL FACE

What can we do?

"Just to be is a blessing, Just to live is Holy." Rabbi Heschel

Early signs/early detection

It is difficult when a loved one gets dementia because of the progressive deterioration of cognitive abilities that we once experienced and used to express our life. In my mother's case, she began to disengage from family activities. Her short-term memory became more difficult to access. She sometimes forgot how to do things like start the car, and she had trouble finding words. These signs were slow and intermittent and because our family was scattered around the country, it was hard for us to get a clear picture together about what was happening. Like many families, we did not know of a family history of dementia and never thought that this was a possibility.

One thing that we face when we see signs of decline is how to approach the topic with sensitivity and love. My sister who is a neurology nurse had been telling me that she thought my mother was "different" for a couple of years, but I think my fear kept me from facing the issue. After a while, however, we did see signs that my mother was having difficulty. When my mother came to visit me for the weekend, it became apparent that she needed help. I called my family and asked them to participate in a conference call, so we could all be on the same page as to how we thought we could help my mother. After the call, we decided that the best thing to do would be to take my mother to Mayo Clinic. With sadness in my heart, I called the clinic and made the appointment. One of my sisters flew down to help with the visit. My family and I talked extensively about how we could help my mother make the adjustments she would need to make and how best to approach this issue with sensitivity and love.

As we age, one of our common fears is that we will lose our independence and our ability to make our own decisions. Some people also fear that they will be thought of as weak or as less of a person. It is very important to remember that many fears come along with the aging process, and to be intentional about how we begin a conversation about aging with our loved one.

Many people try and cope with or hide the disease

For years, we could not speak with my mother over the phone, and we all thought this was because she had a hearing problem. Her father had hearing loss when he got older, so we thought that this was the same kind of thing. What is a probable conclusion when someone finds that they have difficulty hearing over the phone? If, as in my mother's case, the family does not have a history of Alzheimer's or dementia we might conclude that there is a problem with hearing tones over the phone. And because a hearing deficit is acceptable as something that can occur with age, one might continue to let people think that hearing is the problem. That was the case with my mother. It is unfortunate that many people with early-stage dementia attempt to hide their disease, since that is the best time to try and slow its progress.

After my mother was diagnosed with fronto-temporal dementia it became clear that it wasn't a hearing problem that kept us from being able to speak with her on the phone. Instead of a hearing issue, it was that she could not understand what was being said over the phone, because she could not see the person speaking or know the context of the conversation.

When we thought my mother couldn't hear over the phone, we bought her a phone for the hearing impaired. This worked for a while, because she could still read even after she lost most of her verbal communication. Unfortunately this sign of cognitive impairment went undetected for years. Most people try and cover up the signs as long as possible. My mother is a very stoic, intelligent, proud and independent person, and so she was able to cope with her disease a long time without anyone really noticing what was happening.

After she was unable to live at home, I discovered signs of her attempts to cope with this disease. While cleaning out her house, I found that she had put on each hanger in her closet, a complete outfit, including all of the accessories that she would need. She had organized her closet so all she had to do was take out a hanger and she would be "good to go." This took a lot of preparation, but it also took a lot of awareness on her part. I wish she would have told me or anyone that she was having difficulty, so we could begin to help her cope emotionally with this disease and possibly slow its progress with medication.

A change of perception

Many people can and do cover up the initial stages of dementia and Alzheimer's because of the fear and shame attached to these conditions. However, early treatment is imperative if we want to try and slow its progress. Therefore, we need to remove the stigma and shame away from these diseases to be able to help those who have them.

We were all very anxious when we took my mother to the Mayo Clinic. She was very apprehensive about taking the diagnostic tests and it was difficult for me to be with her while she was being tested, because I could tell she thought the tests were degrading. When someone experiences decline, it doesn't mean that they lose sense of who they are and no longer value life. I know that my mother felt embarrassed to be asked questions like, "Who is the president?" and if she could touch her finger to her nose. My mother holds two masters degrees and has been recognized as one of the top teachers in the country. It was a very hard day for her when she had to take these tests, and every time she was asked a question, she would look at me as if to say, "Can you believe that they think I don't know this stuff?" But the real difficulty was that she did not know the answers to some of the questions.

Many of the tests that people are given include very basic questions and this can cause anxiety. My mother was experiencing memory loss and cognitive decline but she still understood the simplicity of the questions and felt that they were demeaning even as she struggled to find the answers.

One significant thing we can do for our loved one is to stay out of our fear so that we do not transfer our emotion on to them. If we focus on our fear for our loved one, it will be difficult for us to stay present and supportive for them. It will also be difficult for everyone involved if we become focused on how we would feel if we were facing this diagnosis. We will experience pain and grief, so it is important to work through and allow ourselves to experience our feelings, so that we can be present for our loved one when they need us. We also need to find and use a good support system to help us process our experience, while remembering that our loved one needs us to be fully present and supportive as well.

After my mother was given her verbal tests at Mayo Clinic, we went down to get an MRI taken of her brain. The MRI worried me because I knew that the pictures would give us irrefutable proof of her disease. I sat with her as she waited for her MRI and helped her dress after the test was finished. When she returned to the changing area, my mother was smiling. She was smiling because she wanted to convince both me and herself that she had "passed" the tests. It was very sad for me to hear her tell me that the technician told her that she had "done very well," because I knew she wanted this to mean that there was nothing wrong with the images on the scan. My mother knew what she was being tested for, but she did not want it to be acknowledged or confirmed. I couldn't blame her for those feelings, because I did not want to see what the tests would reveal either. I am sure she shared my thought that, once there was a diagnosis, there was no more room for hope...or is there? I have since learned that... *It all depends on for what we are hoping*.

Hope of a new possibility

"There is in all visible things...a hidden wholeness." Thomas Merton

If our hope is that the dementia can be reversed and that our loved one will live life as they always have, we will be disappointed because as yet no cure exists. But this isn't to say that will always be the case. In the future perhaps a cure for this disease will be discovered. Until that day, we can find hope in something that goes beyond a cure, which is the knowledge that a person with dementia can continue to thrive, be in relationship, and maintain a sense of peace in his or her life. This can happen when we take an active role in turning a possibility in to a reality. In order for this to occur, we must let go of what our culture has taught us about life.

Because dementia has become known as "the long goodbye", our focus has been on the slow decline of our loved one. This comes from focusing on the departure of the societal and cultural pieces that make up the identity of an individual. "The long goodbye" creates an image of a person who is slowly going away, and for the family, it is a slow and painful path to saying goodbye. *But this statement creates a sense of helplessness and grief for families and places the focus on dying rather than living.*

I have always had a very adverse reaction to this statement, because while I know that my mother is slowly losing abilities and no longer would be defined by society as she once was while healthy. Her life is still beautiful and vibrant. While it is true that people with dementia lose many abilities, labeling someone's life as "the long goodbye" distracts us from the life being lived in the present moment.

Cognitive impairment can decrease the ability to perform many functions. Some of the most difficult challenges for the family members and loved ones to experience are the inability to retrieve memory, a lack of communication, a lack of recognition, and a lack of perceived emotion. A loss of memory and recognition feels like a loss of connection for everyone. Memory is one of the things that hold us together in space and time; it keeps us grounded and connected to life and to those around us. It is often devastating for families when the person with dementia no longer recognizes them. This can feel as if we are no longer significant in our loved one's life. Remember, the pain involved in memory loss can go both ways. It is also frustrating for many people with dementia to not know someone who comes to visit. I see people with this disease become very frustrated and sometimes sad when they have to be reminded that someone who they think they do not know is actually a significant person in their life.

Some people with dementia experience decreased affect and display little or no facial expression, which can become very difficult for family members and loved ones, since we rely on these expressions as part of our nonverbal communication. We know someone is happy to see us when they smile. We know that we have been recognized when someone's facial expression changes as we go into their room or enter their energetic space. It can feel harder for us to connect without these verbal and nonverbal cues in general, and when the loss of these cues is due to cognitive disease, it brings with it an added sense of grief.

WHAT IS POSSIBLE?

The journey

"When we complete the journey to our own heart, we will find ourselves in the hearts of everyone else." Father Thomas Keating

Beyond limitations

We possess a unique ability to go beyond our perceived limitations. Every journey we take begins with the first step, and the journey of moving past the limits of traditional communication begins with how we interpret the different stages of this disease and where we look for signs of life. What we focus on has a significant impact on what we find. If we focus on the disease and the limitations, that is what we will see. If we look at one another with new awareness and focus on the beauty of our eternal spirit, we will see the beauty of life lived in the present moment.

The greatest gift we can give our loved one is to create and channel positive energy to them. I believe that it is my responsibility to find what will enhance positive energy for my mother and foster it. To do this I have taught myself to move beyond my traditional ideas about what is positive. We can all go beyond these traditional ideas, and it only requires us to free our loved one from their past identity and create new possibilities for them. We can do this by accepting that even though their past abilities used to serve them well, they are not necessary any longer. More importantly, these abilities are not necessary for their lives to be beautiful.

Creative communication

My mother, a former English teacher with two Master's degrees, was a very articulate person. Her frontal lobe dementia has left her unable to speak. For me, as her daughter, I believe that it is necessary and possible to find new ways to communicate and to acknowledge this communication as something positive. I think that the difficult part for many people is to believe that these new ways of communicating can be meaningful and valid. Communication is not only an exchange of ideas and information; it is also a form of connection and an exchange of energy. Losing the ability to find and use words was very frustrating and scary to my mother as her disease progressed. It became difficult for her when someone spoke to her beyond a simple sentence, because she could not follow what they were saying. Even now she seems to get frustrated and often walks away when someone says more than one sentence to her. However, my mother does show us that she is open to and will participate in other forms of communication and other ways to connect.

Even though my mother responds to verbal directions and simple questions, she does not speak. For example, when asked if she wants a drink, she might nod or pick up her glass. She seems to get upset if spoken to at length. Therefore I have found it helpful to use an object, sign language, music, or a picture to communicate with her. While visiting her one day, I found an abacus on one of the tables where she lives and decided to see if I could use it as a way to engage and connect with my mother. I moved half of the pieces of the abacus to either side and then slid the abacus over to her. She looked at it, moved all the pieces over to the same side and slid the abacus back over to me. This simple game gives me another way to interact with my mother without her getting frustrated. It helps me feel connected with her when she looks up and smiles as she pushes the abacus back to me. My nieces and I call this the "abacus game," and my mother sits for hours playing it with us. If I were to place a negative judgment on playing the abacus game, I would lose a significant opportunity to interact with my mother. Judging ourselves or another person halts our possibility to be fully engaged in life.

How can we be safe for our loved one?

"He who wants to do good knocks at the gate. He who loves finds the gate open." Rabindranath Tagore

Beyond frustration

We often feel powerless when a loved one gets sick or goes through a difficult situation. We feel powerless because we think that nothing we do can help fix or change what is happening. But there are things we can do to help improve the life of a loved one in significant ways. One of the things that we can do is be a "safe" person with whom they can express openly how they are feeling and what they are experiencing. How we interact with a person who has a debilitating disease helps remove feelings of shame, improves their sense of self worth, and can help plant the seed of hope.

Even though many things associated with dementia and Alzheimer's lead to frustration, we must remember that how we react and relate to and with one another is important in any personal relationship. When someone has dementia, how we relate to them can have a significant impact on their quality of life. If we treat a person with dementia as if they are a cause of frustration to us or if we begin to act as if they are less of a person because they have this disease, we will diminish their quality of life.

One thing we experience when a loved one has dementia is the opportunity to listen to the same stories over and over again. We also find that we repeat conversations.

It can be frustrating when our loved one forgets seeing us from day to day or gets angry at us for not visiting more often when we were just over yesterday. We can find ourselves in a tricky situation when our mother, father, or spouse comes over to mow our lawn or feed our pets and begins to have trouble with their memory. Maybe our spouse or parent starts calling us during the day to ask a question about how or what to feed the pets or maybe they are getting lost going to the grocery store. Many of us have responded in this situation by reminding our father that he feeds the dog all the time and should know where the food is kept or we tell our mother that the store is right down the road where it has always been. But the questions we should be asking in these situations and the reminders we give need to be addressed to ourselves.

A different response

Some helpful questions that we can ask ourselves in these situations are: "Is a story only important or worth our time if it is a new story?" And... "What is the point of telling someone experiencing memory loss that they have already told us something?" Just taking the time to think about what is happening before we respond out of frustration is beneficial. It is helpful for both of us if we remember that a person who forgets simple tasks and retells stories probably already knows that there is a change in their ability to remember. One of the most supportive things we can do is to remember that this is a frightening, uncertain, and painful time for everyone involved. A positive and life-affirming response to our loved one's difficulties does not include reminding them that they are forgetting or show that they are causing us frustration. Remember that change creates fear in most people and the changes in memory require that we have compassion for one another.

What we can do when our loved one forgets how to do simple tasks is to put up labels, instructions, and pictures to help them remember. This will help our loved one continue to feel helpful and engaged. I have found that many people in early stages of this disease know that they are forgetful and that they cannot form thoughts. One woman I used to visit would say to me, "It's crazy! I just don't know anymore." She knew that she had trouble forming thoughts and was very aware of her cognitive decline. Pointing out these lapses can actually create distance between you and your loved one. Of course we cannot pretend that the signs do not exist, but we can be intentional about how and when we begin to have a conversation about it.

Beyond fear

Cognitive decline is a very sensitive subject and needs to be addressed with care and compassion.

When we begin to think about having a conversation with a family member regarding a decline in any ability, what is most important is that we create a safe environment. A safe environment requires emotional, spiritual, and physical safety. It also requires that each person involved in the conversation is "safe" for the person experiencing cognitive decline. Being "safe" for another person means that we can hear what the other person is saying without judgment, measuring, or labeling. To be able to really hear what another person is saying to us requires that we detach our ego from the conversation. This means we will not be connected to the content or to the outcome of the conversation. If we enter in to this conversation with the intent that there will be a specific outcome, we will not be able to listen with compassion, because we will be focused on achieving that outcome rather than listening to our loved one. Remember that this is a very frightening time for our loved one and, although we need to make sure that we are doing everything to ensure their physical safety, their emotional and spiritual safety is just as important.

When we begin to have a conversation about cognitive decline, it is normal for our loved one to deny a problem and even to get angry with us. If they express anger, try to focus on hearing and speaking to the emotion. If our loved one is angry, we can de-escalate their anger just by letting them know that we have heard them. How we feel about the anger and what we think about the anger is not the point in this conversation. Do not respond to the emotion with judgment; rather, respond with understanding by acknowledging whatever they are feeling. When we acknowledge the emotion without judgment, we can then move on to finding the reason for the emotion.

Beyond words

Hearing another person is one of the best gifts that we can give. However, most of us think that if we let someone know that we have heard them, we are essentially saying that we are in agreement. While it may feel this way, it is not necessarily the case. We can hear what another person is saying, even if we do not agree with what they say or understand their point of view. Hearing one another has a tremendous potential for healing. Truly hearing another person validates them and their experience. Being able to hear another person is a gift that we can give that can help heal the spirit. Hearing one another is essential. It needs to be our primary goal when we have a conversation with our loved one.

The best possible solutions come from hearing one another

Imagine how it would feel if you were about to have a conversation with someone or a group of people who disagreed with you or acted as if you were "less than." Generally in this situation we might feel anxiety, frustration, or anger. We might also feel as though we need to defend ourselves and who we are. It is very difficult to have a discussion when we are feeling these kinds of emotions. Our emotional response comes into play when we feel who we are and how we live is being questioned. It is impossible to work with another person or engage in open dialogue when we feel that we are being made wrong or when we are making someone else wrong. The way to create possibilities for solutions with another person or group of people therefore comes from the ability to hear one another.

Hearing one another requires that individuals act with intention, which takes practice and patience. We tend to think that we are listening when another person is speaking. However, what most of us are doing is *waiting* for our own opportunity to speak. This has to do with trying to get our ideas across in such a way that the other person will agree with us. But if the other person has a different set of ideas then, as we try and convince them to see our point of view, we are also telling them that their point of view is wrong.

How many times have we caught ourselves waiting for the other person to pause or take a breath so that we can begin to speak? When we are only concerned about stating our ideas, rather than listening, conversations become more of a pushing back and forth than an open exchange of ideas. A dialogue can only happen when there is the intention of actually hearing what one another has to say. The important part of having a dialogue is listening for and hearing the message the other person is trying to convey.

Hearing our loved one

When we are able to hear what another person is saying, he or she feels supported and validated, which leads to a more productive conversation. For example, if we are talking with our loved one about recent memory loss, it is common for the person to become defensive, angry, or even deny that there is any validity to what we are saying. People who are angry often lash out with angry words. The angry words are actually used to try to get the other person to "back up," creating space so they feel safer. It helps when we do not get caught up in what is being said, but instead try and understand *why* it is being said. Hurtful words are often fueled by pain. If we do hear the emotion and speak to it, our loved will know that we are actually listening.

We might hear our loved one telling us that we are meddling in their life. Instead of responding to that statement, look for its source. Meddling is usually thought of as getting into another person's business and perhaps even trying to make decisions for that person without their permission. Therefore when our mother, father, spouse, or sibling starts to talk about meddling, it may come from fear of losing their independence. Staying independent for an older person is very important. If we hear a statement about our meddling, we can ask our loved one what we both could do to help them remain as independent as they can for as long as possible. A question like this helps us check that we have heard the emotion and also enables us to validate their concerns.

Hearing one another

By hearing the whole message, whether there is a concern, or fear, etc., we de-escalate the emotion which will allow us to be able to speak to the issue. By letting our loved one know that we have heard their fear, regardless of whether we agree or feel the fear is based in reality, the fear will diminish significantly. We will then be able to have a conversation about how to best move forward so that our loved one feels safe, cared for, and happy. By de-escalating the emotion, we are able to enter into a partnership for solutions. Three ways to know that we have heard someone correctly include: when the person tells us we have done so, when there is a drop in emotional energy, and when the other person does not repeat themselves. I always know that I have not heard someone when the person speaking feels the need to repeat what they have said.

The key to hearing another person is to listen to both the message and the emotion. Remember, the message is not always exactly what is being said. Hearing does not mean that we "mirror" back word for word what the person has just said to us. Mirroring can be a way of pretending to hear and sometimes feels unauthentic to the other person. We all know that very often what we say and what we mean are not the same. Listen to your loved one. Can you hear the message behind their words? Can you speak to their fear, frustration, anger, or pain? When we are able to hear one another, we become a safe person and only then we can help the healing process begin.

Putting our baggage aside

Our own baggage can hinder our ability to listen to others. Before we can be present for another person who is grieving a loss, for example, we must first understand how we feel about grief and loss. Our own emotions can distract us and, if we want to be fully present for another person, we need to be able to deal with our own emotions or at least able to set them aside so they do not enter into our conversation. It is common to project on to another person, our own unresolved issues. Projection can cause conflict in an already difficult situation. It is okay if we realize we need a little room to process our feelings about what is happening with our loved one. And it is healthier for everyone involved when we are honest about where we are and how much we are able to be involved in their care and life. This will allow us to have compassion for ourselves, for our loved one with the disease, and for our family members. Compassion is being able to understand another person's experience without becoming part of it.

Dementia affects the entire family

When a loved one has dementia, the entire family is affected, and we all need to give one another and ourselves the time and grace to go through our own process, whatever that might look like. There may be different roles that each person is willing and able to take on when a love one has dementia. Some of us will be able to be very involved in their care and life, while others will not. It is important that family members understand and accept that we will all deal with this disease differently and try to give one another the grace to do so. We will only create more pain if we judge our brothers and sisters, mothers, and fathers; because we think they should be or do something differently.

Grieving

Grieving is okay. I have grieved for a future that will not happen, for family events that my mother would have loved, for the loss of a beloved grandmother for her grandchildren, and for how she would have loved to and expected to be involved in their lives. It saddens me to know how proud she would have been that her daughter- in-law received the "Teacher of the Year Award," since my mother was also a teacher. I know that the world has lost the chance to be affected by a wonderfully compassionate person who, when she retired wanted to hold babies in the ICU and to feed and work with the homeless.

It is important to honor and work through the emotions that we have when our loved one has dementia. One thing that is helpful is to work on our own issues about self identity and how we evaluate one another. We must understand what dementia means to us before we try and connect with someone who has this disease. We can be a safe person when we do not try to change what the other person is feeling or try to fix the situation. Being diagnosed with dementia is a frightening experience. If we can hear our loved ones fears, they can become less afraid. Often we are uncomfortable with how another person is feeling, and we try to get them to change. But being a safe person means allowing another person to experience their life without judgment and without focusing on our need to feel comfortable.

Family dynamics

"We are only as strong as the support that we give to one another." Linn Possell

We have all heard of the line that is used with teams and group activities: "You are only as strong as your weakest link." That might work with a link of chain, but it does not work with people, because people are infinitely varied; and are multidimensional. Although we may have a particular weakness in one area, we probably have many strengths in other areas. Instead, we need a phrase that can help us understand how important we are to one another. "We are only as strong as the support that we give to one another." This is important to remember because we all have different abilities, life situations, gifts, and limitations. Family dynamics work better when we remember that we are only as strong as the support that we give to one another.

Remember too that if we cannot be the primary caregiver of our loved one, it is vital that we support the person who is. Being a caregiver is a very stressful and lonely role at times. Even if your loved one is in a full-care facility, it is important that all of the members of the family participate in their loved one's life in the best way that each one can.

Beyond the past

Everyone is in a different place in their life and this will affect how we respond to the situations we face and the experiences we have. Therefore, each of us will respond differently to the fact that our loved one has dementia. As with anything in our lives, our history with our loved one and our hope for the future will influence how we deal with this situation. However, only we can decide whether these things are positive influences or negative influences.

A difficult past

If we have had a challenging relationship with our loved one prior to the onset of their disease, it may be more difficult to think that our interaction will be positive. Maybe we were hurt by the person who now has dementia. Perhaps they did something that caused us pain or were less-involved or supportive in our lives than we would have hoped. Maybe we were not able to resolve these feelings of anger, hurt, or disappointment. What do we do when we find ourselves faced with a situation where there is no chance to resolve these issues? Is there a way to let go of the negative energy of a difficult past relationship?

Holding on to negative energy can become debilitating and can even control our lives. However, we can release ourselves from this negative energy and allow resolution to take place if this is what we chose. Resolution and the possibility for creating a new relationship will come if we chose to practice forgiveness. When we forgive ourselves or another person, we let go of the negative energy and the emotion connected to that situation. Forgiveness is a way of freeing ourselves of pain and negativity that often hold us back from living our life freely.

We all want to feel as if we have the power to make decisions that will impact our lives, but when we harbor resentment and anger toward someone or even toward ourselves, that resentment and anger controls our life. When we are free of these emotions and negative energy we are empowered to live freely and fully.

Forgiveness frees us from the bonds of negative energy. This does not mean forgetting what has happened in the past. However, in order to be free, we have to let go of negative energy. Sometimes we find it hard to forgive because it feels as if we are letting the other person off the hook for what they have done in the past. We don't usually want to let that person off the hook or say what they did was "okay." We want the other person to acknowledge that what they did was wrong or hurtful. Most of the time it is important to us that we feel vindicated, as if we are right and justified for our feelings. Simply put...we want justice.

The soul does not carry emotional baggage

We have been taught that justice means that someone has to pay for their actions and we feel even more justified when they admit their guilt. The situation that we have with dementia, which might be hard to come to terms with for many of us, is that the person with this disease is essentially freed from their past. With a loss of memory comes the release of past pain. Our souls do not carry emotional baggage. It may take some work to come to terms with this idea. Until we can deal with this reality, however, we are the only ones who will be hurt by the situation. If we find ourselves feeling upset that the person with dementia or Alzheimer's cannot either apologize or take responsibility for their actions, it is a good indication that we need to work on forgiveness.

Forgiveness will help free our lives and may enable us to see the other person differently. When we make the conscious choice to let go of the negative energy we carry with us, we can find forgiveness and live in the present moment. Forgiveness creates healing because it allows life to move freely toward love and love is the highest frequency of energy there is. It can free us from the baggage of our past and open us to joy.

Beyond out-dated beliefs about justice

It seems as if our beliefs about justice are major blocks to forgiveness. Our wisdom teachers, however, taught us that there is another form of justice. Jesus called it the "justice of God." This justice is not about retribution, but equality. This justice has nothing to do with being good or bad, right or wrong. A just world allows for everyone to have an equal chance at life. A just world is not a world where people are measured and labeled and where we cause pain to one another. An equal chance at life does not mean that everything has to be equal for everyone, but it does mean that everyone has an equal opportunity to experience life in its fullest form. The justice of God requires our participation. Holding on to past hurts or basing our happiness on whether someone else changes how they are living or demanding retribution is not part of God's justice.

When we hold on to the need to be vindicated for something that has happened in the past, we create an obstacle for life in the present. If we base our ability or decision to move forward with our life on the willingness of another person to take responsibility or to change, then we are putting a barrier in front of us that only we can move. Forgiveness means that we free ourselves and the other person from something negative. For life to move toward healing and wholeness, we must find ways to forgive one another.

We also need to find ways to forgive ourselves. Maybe we did not have the best relationship with our family member who has dementia. Regardless of what has happened in the past, we have the power to reclaim our life and reclaim the possibilities for ourselves and for our loved one. There are many opportunities for feelings of guilt and pain to arise when we deal with dementia. Some family members are able to visit and be involved in care and others are not. Remember that judgment is an obstacle to love. Love and forgiveness are equivalent and together they can free us from the past so that we are able to embrace life.

When we practice forgiveness, it is as if we remove an added weight we have carried around that has prevented us from experiencing the fullness of life. Negative energy and holding on to pain or anger stop us from connecting to our spirit and the spirits of others.

A HOLISTIC APPROACH

Energy

"Energy is a circle. It returns to you" Karyn Mitchell

Growth comes from connecting to the source of life which some people call God and is universally called Spirit. Spirit is the eternal energy that permeates and gives life to all things. When we judge ourselves or someone else, we stop our spiritual, emotional, and intellectual growth because judgment creates negative energy. Energy is drawn to and connects with similar energy and so, when we devalue one another in any way, we send negative energy out in to the world. Mother Theresa once said, "If you judge people, you have no time to love them." It only takes a moment to refocus our thoughts so that we can focus on what is positive and bring positive energy to one another. If I focus on what someone can no longer do, whether that is reading, speaking, doing simple tasks, or even remembering, I am focusing on *my perception* of what is lacking. However, if I focus on the reality of the present moment, I am able to celebrate life as it is.

When we are with our loved one, it is always good to make an assessment of our own energy before we enter into their presence. It is good to check our energy because positive energy sustains life and has a nourishing effect on us. The immune system is a good example of what negative energy and stress can do to life. When we feel stress, our cortisol levels increase and our immune system's ability to help us sustain life decreases. Excess cortisol is toxic to our bodies. A minute of stress can depress the immune system for hours before it can come back into balance.

What do you tell yourself about Alzheimer's and dementia? I recently heard someone say that their father was a victim of this disease. I have heard other people call a person with dementia "poor." Even though it may be said out of sympathy, this statement focuses on the disease. By focusing on the disease we create a sense of a disvalued state of being. What language do you use when you think or talk about dementia?

Sympathy and compassion

Sympathy and compassion are two very different things. Webster's dictionary defines sympathy as "an association or relationship between persons or things wherein whatever affects one similarly affects the other."When we have sympathy for an individual with dementia, it is difficult to make a connection with that person, because our focus is on the disease. When we focus on the disease, we tend to project our emotions on to our loved one. By projecting, we think about how we would feel if we had this disease or how we imagine the emotions that a person has who is aware of their dementia. Of course no one wants to get dementia, but people with cognitive impairment usually do not stay aware of their disease for a long period of time. At some point they will move beyond the awareness that they have the disease. Once they have moved past the initial stage of knowing that they are declining, they are not necessarily aware of their loss of cognitive function. Therefore they do not feel the grief that we may feel when we see them decline. To feel sympathy for someone with dementia does not benefit either person.

Empathy is different. Empathy involves being able to enter in to another person's experience so that we can, on some level, understand what they are feeling. Empathy is a way of attuning ourselves to another person and this leads to compassion, in which we are led to take action to help improve that person's experience. In other words, compassion means to "feel with" and to use this connection as the impetus for action.

It is important to really try and understand our loved one's experience. If we observe a person who has dementia, it is possible to learn the signs that can help us understand how they are feeling and what they are experiencing. We cannot take action that will help our mother, father, spouse, or sibling, if we do not understand what they are experiencing. Some of the signs to look for include body language and their level of agitation or contentment. There are also physical signs such as blood pressure and temperature that can be signs of discomfort. For example, high blood pressure in someone that does not usually have it can be a sign of discomfort.

At the facility where my mother lives they are very observant for signs that might indicate a change in the disease or a change in a resident's experience. For example, one day the nurse called me to tell me that they were concerned because my mother was "leaning" to one side more than usual. The fact that my mother was leaning was a sign that she was in pain and after a urine test they found out that she had a Urinary Tract Infection. As we look for such signs, we might need to change our way of looking for clues about life. The usual signs and ways of communicating we use with one another often times no longer work for those who have dementia.

Suffering

"Peace comes from within. Do not seek it without."
The Buddha

Beyond "should"

Many things in life are hard to bear and yet, in the midst of all of these circumstances, we can also find much to embrace. Life holds within it endless joy and beauty. We cannot choose the circumstances that we face in life, but we can choose how we will walk through them. While we make the choice as to how we respond and engage any situation, we must be patient with ourselves and with others in our life experiences.

We are in control of our experiences and can choose to see and embrace the life that is present even in the midst of pain and disappointment. But before we can do this, we need to acknowledge our pain and grief and work on moving through these emotions, because if we deny our grief, we also deny our joy. Once we have worked through our grief, it becomes possible to look for the sources of joy.

Some of the things that I miss about my mother are taking walks with her, working in the garden, and listening to her play the guitar. But I continue to find joy in the fact that I still get to hear her laugh and hold her hand.

Connection happens when we let go of our idea of limitation. With dementia can come a loss of memory of our shared history and the loss of recognition of our loved ones. Even with memory, it is still possible to build meaningful connections. In order to be fully present and connected, we need to take the time to face some difficult questions. These include questions such as:

- "What does it mean to me when my loved one forgets that I am his or her son, daughter, brother, sister, spouse, etc?"

- Does this invalidate our history or our relationship?

- Does it mean that we are no longer important to that person?

There is usually a sense of grief that accompanies our loved one's loss of memory, and it is important to acknowledge whatever emotions come up for us during this time of processing. The connections we make in the future with our loved one depend on our ability to work through our emotions.

Obviously we experience a whole host of emotions when someone we love has Alzheimer's and or dementia, and it is important to acknowledge and sit with these emotions until we can work through them. What helps this shift happen is when we are patient with ourselves. It will not help if we try and deny or distance ourselves from our experience. It is also important to remember that whatever we experience is valid, and that we cannot compare our experience with anyone else's. We all respond differently to situations in our lives, so everyone involved in this process needs to be given the room and the permission to acknowledge, feel, and process their emotions.

The Buddha teaches that we create our own suffering, and this is created by our desire. Moving toward or away from something is the source of suffering. If we want our loved one to be something that they will never be, then we will create suffering for ourselves. Suffering does not allow us to see or connect to the life of our loved one. Suffering is a distraction that separates us from those around us.

Suffering comes from our belief that reality should be different than it is. If I believe that my mother should not have dementia, and if I make that thought the only way that I will be happy, I have just created my own suffering. The reality is that she does have dementia. While it is important that I work through my stages of grief, it is unhealthy for everyone involved if I stay stuck in my grief and continue to want reality to be different. When I do not accept reality, then I cannot live in what "is" and so I cannot live a compassionate life. If my need for my mother to say my name outweighs the fact that she recognizes me as someone significant in her life, then I will suffer. If, however, I accept that she may not know that I am her daughter and that she is unable to say my name, I am free to celebrate what she "is" able to do. What "is', at least for the present, is that she recognizes me as someone significant in her life. I find joy in that recognition and awareness and celebrate that she remains connected to me. I also know that this may change at some point, as her disease progresses.

Our suffering comes from our need for, our desire of, and our choice to hold on to something that is no longer reality. Healing for ourselves comes when we release ourselves from these needs and release our loved one from being responsible for our happiness. When we have a loved one with dementia, we have a choice. We can suffer with the belief that something has to be different to preserve our happiness, or we can celebrate the life being lived. If our goal is for our loved one to experience fullness of life, then we need to change our expectations. To do this, we can learn what fullness of life is for that person and help them experience this.

Beyond suffering

My mother has taught me that fullness of life means to live in the reality of what "is" rather than what "should be." It is possible to find joy in very simple things, and when we spend time with people who have dementia, they can be powerful reminders of this. Suffering happens when we refuse to accept what is, and think that it should be different, or when we make our happiness contingent on something else being different. Rather than saying, "I want my mother to be able to recognize me," try and change the statement to, "I want to be able to recognize my mother." Recognize her for who she is now, recognize her spirit that continues to live and find expression in this world. We will be able to recognize the spirit when we see our mother, father, or spouse as whole and beautiful just the way they are in the present moment.

Our story

One way to stop our suffering is to focus on celebrating our life stories, both past and present. Our life stories are important to us because they help us see where we have been and where we are. Stories help point to possible futures. They are also important because they help us share our experiences with one another. Storytelling is a way to pass on our history and find common experiences that can help create significant bonds.

When someone we love dies, we usually gather and tell stories about their life. Remembering is another form of meeting, and through telling stories we feel a sense of connection with the one we remember and with those around us. During our times of grief, part of our healing process begins with telling our stories. This is also important for the families of people who have dementia. If our loved one happens to live in a full-care facility, it is helpful for the caregivers to know his or her story, because it helps caregivers know that person on a more intimate level and helps them connect with that person. Telling our stories and sharing things about our loved one is essential to the families, because we want people to know them as we do. We are often proud of their accomplishments and of the way they lived, and want to celebrate what makes them unique.

"The long goodbye", however, becomes a reality if we hold on to our story of the past and refuse to let the story continue in the present. When we find ourselves attached to the story, we become attached to the past, and what we focus on may not be possible in the present. We suffer because we want the story to remain the same. If we need the story to continue the way it has in the past, then it is difficult for us to embrace the expression of life that exists in the present moment. The story is still true, our loved one did express themselves as an artist or musician, displayed courage and patience, gave to charity, sang in the choir, etc. But if our need for them to continue to find expression like this is greater than our acceptance of their new expression and this new chapter in their story, we will find it difficult to connect with them in their present life. When the story becomes a measurement, when it is the only thing that brings value to life, then our story becomes a barrier to the spirit.

What gives life purpose?

"The fullness of joy is to behold God in everything." Julian of Norwich

The belief that we have to do something measurable is a stumbling block over which many of us fall. We are constantly judging whether our life has "measured up to" some idea of what it is supposed to be or whether we have done anything worthy enough to call our life valuable. The idea of a "purposeful life" is misleading. There have been a lot of books published that perpetuate the belief that our lives need to have a purpose in order for them to have any worth or value. It seems as if we have bought in to the belief that life needs a special purpose for it to have any relevance or meaning. There are many people who care more about their purpose than they do about other people.

I believe that the meaning of life is to live it. Living life with consideration and awareness of others and other life around us. Living life does not mean that we should be stepping on and over anyone else while we try to climb to the top of whatever ladder we have chosen to climb. Nor does it mean that we should not care about future generations and the future of our world. The idea of living a life that has a purpose does not ensure that we will live in harmony with others. The idea that our life has to have a purpose comes from our need to feed our ego, because it reinforces our need to be viable and valuable to society.

Thinking that we must have a stated purpose in life is often distracting and can actually hinder us from finding what is meaningful in our lives. This happens because the idea of purpose focuses us on our need to build our self esteem and our desire to feed our ego. Our lack of self esteem and our attachment to ego come from our culture and our belief that we must prove ourselves worthy. It comes from looking to outside sources for approval and help defining who we are as people. If instead we believed what we are taught by all of the wisdom teachers, we would realize that we are all worthy and valuable. Mathew Fox, in his book, *Original Blessing*, writes about this inherent worth. We are worthy and valuable because we have been given life, and life is sacred.

One summer while I watched my three-year-old niece play on the beach, I was struck with a new understanding of purpose. I watched for hours as she went to the water, filled her bucket with water, brought it back to where she was digging, put sand into the bucket, and then poured it all out. What was the purpose of her actions? They didn't make sense to me, but as I watched her, what *did* make sense was that she found joy in her experience.

What makes my niece's experience any less than mine or yours? Although we may interact with people, work, and accomplish things that may be more highly valued in society than she can do at age three, her life has as much worth as any other. My niece's experience was one of joy and contentment, which we all can experience when we live in the present moment without attachment to our ego and our need for outside approval.

One day as I spent time with my mother while she was still in the beginning stages of this disease, the mail came to her house. My mother always had subscriptions to magazines, and some of them came in the mail that day. I remember watching my mother as she sat down on the couch with the magazines and began to randomly tear out pages. She continued to do this until almost every page was gone. As I watched her, I kept asking her why she was tearing out the pages, to which I got no response. And then it dawned on me that it didn't really matter if it made sense to me why she was tearing out the pages. What mattered was that it appeared as if my mother was doing something that had a purpose for her; it was an activity that she could actually do. I remember saying out loud to myself, "It doesn't matter why she's tearing up the magazine. What matters is that she wants to do it."

"People with Alzheimer's and dementia can thrive."
Jennifer D'Eugenio, Alzheimer's Resource Center of
Connecticut

Facility or home?

With a supportive and loving environment, people
with dementia can and do find contentment and
joy. The key is to find an environment that has the
philosophy and culture that all life is sacred and
that has the kind of staff who believe that people
with dementia can thrive.

It is often traumatic for families to think about
having their mother, father, spouse, etc. live in a
full-care facility. We have difficulty imagining that
the quality of life is the same in a facility as it is in
our home, but if we find the right one, it can
create a wonderful opportunity for healing. This
healing can affect both the person with dementia
and the family. One of the first things that we need
to do is allow ourselves to be free of the guilt that
comes along with a decision to place a loved one in
a full-care facility. Our guilt usually comes from the
promise that we make, to never place our loved
one in an institution.

Years before my mother was diagnosed with
dementia, we had the same conversation over and
over again. She would ask what would happen to
her if she were to become ill when she got older.
And I would answer that I would take care of her. I
repeatedly told my mother than she would live with
me and I promised never to put her in a nursing

home. I told her I would always find a way to take care of her and begged her not to worry.

I promised to always take care of my mother and I struggled to fulfill that promise when I was told that the best thing for her was a full-care facility. Our family worked with an expert in dementia care who knew my mother's situation. One day when I called her regarding something that had happened, this expert told me that the best thing for my mother was to move into a full-care facility. Although I did not want to hear this and argued my point for keeping my mother at home, I knew in the back of my mind that I needed to trust the professionals who knew a lot more than I did about this disease and about how to care for people with this disease.

I struggled because I thought that by having my mother live in a facility and not in my home with me, I would not be able to keep my promise. But with the help of a support group, I realized that I made this promise when my mother was well, when dementia was a disease completely foreign to my family. I was prepared to keep my mother in my home if she had cancer like my grandmother or if she was unable to care for herself because of the normal decline that accompanies the aging process. However, dementia was one variable among others that I never imagined would happen.

Finding appropriate care

When we were trying to care for my mother in the home, we encountered many unexpected obstacles. My mother began to eat inedible objects, we had to put everything she could choke on out of her reach. We had to lock the refrigerator, because she was always seeking food and putting too much in her mouth and then choking on it. When we tried to take her to a day-care facility, we were told she was not appropriate for the facility because she was an "elopement risk." It seemed as if no one wanted to help us nor could they understand my mother and her needs. My mother was not trying to "escape" the facility; she just did not understand that she needed to stay inside. My mother always loved to walk outside so when she saw a door, she opened the door and walked out. But this made her an "elopement risk," not appropriate for a day program.

Sometimes the task of finding the right care for our loved one seems too difficult. We tried several different programs. None of them seemed to work for my mother, or we were told that she was not appropriate. These programs were costly to our family, both monetarily and emotionally. There were many obstacles in our way to finding the best solution for my mother, and it sometimes felt as if the easiest thing to do would be to give up. The one thing that kept me going was my promise that I would always take care of her, and so whatever obstacle came our way, we chose to get over, around or through it for her sake.

I made my mother a promise with complete honesty and commitment. My support group also helped remind me that in my promise, I had also made a covenant with my mother that I would always take care of her. And therefore, she lives in an environment that is beyond what my family could provide in our home, where she is surrounded by people who help her live a joyful and contented life. I was able to keep my promise to her by being persistent and by trusting the professionals in dementia care who helped us find her the most appropriate environment in which to live.

Helping our loved ones adjust

Even if we are able to find a great facility for our loved one, it is very difficult to leave them for the first time. While it was very difficult caring for my mother at home, we still did not fully understand all of the implications of her disease. When my family and I did decide to try having my mother live in a facility designed to care for people with dementia, we chose an assisted-living facility for memory care. It was so traumatic for us when we took her to the facility the first day, because we had just begun to process the fact that my mother would not be living at home anymore. However, we tried our best to help her adjust to her new environment. I stayed with my mother for the entire day, participating in activities and eating with her. At lunch she looked at me and asked to go home, and I thought that my heart would break. I looked at her and said, "This is your home now, Mom." She understood what I was saying, and her eyes filled with tears. I kept telling her that she would be okay, as I wished with my whole heart that I could instead take her home.

As my partner stayed with my mother, my sister and I went up to speak to the administrator and head nurse. There they told us that the best thing to do would be to leave for a while so they could help my mother adjust to her new surroundings. The staff instructed my partner to leave while my mother was occupied, so that she would not become upset. It continues to be a painful memory when she had to turn her back on my mother and slip out the door.

We were only at my sister's house for an hour, when we received a call from the facility telling us that I needed to come back immediately. When I entered the facility, I saw the administrator in the lobby using a walkie talkie. From the balcony of the front lobby, she called down to me asking if I had seen my mother. Of course I hadn't seen my mother! I had just gotten out of the car, and the memory-care unit was a locked facility. Be careful if you are told that a facility is locked. This unit did have locked doors, but if someone pushed on them for any length of time, they would open. The staff was on high alert because my mother had done just that. She had gone to the door, pushed on it, and walked out.

In the back of the unit there were windows and some of the parking lot was visible from these windows. My mother had seen a car like hers, opened the door, and went out to the parking lot. As I ran around the facility looking for her, I found her near a white Jeep Cherokee like the one she used to drive.

Well, that was all the staff needed. My mother was labeled an "elopement risk" and deemed inappropriate for the facility. We asked if she could stay there until we figured out what to do next, and they said my mother could stay if I stayed with her. My sister, partner, and brother-in-law all took shifts so we could stay with my mother around the clock and keep her from "eloping" again. My partner and I spent the night with my mother, a difficult and painful night for all of us. She would not go in to her room or lie down on her bed. We walked for hours, and every time we walked past my mother's room, I would point to it and tell her that that it was her room. We did get her to lie down on one of the couches in the activity room for about 20 twenty minutes, but then we were up and walking again.

I finally got my mother to lie down in her bed around 1:00 a.m., but that was probably because she was exhausted. However, she would only lie in her bed if I sat next to her and held her hand. I sat there through the night, holding my mother's hand, so that she could sleep. My partner sat by the door to make sure she did not get up without anyone noticing. It broke my heart to see my mother in this situation and to watch her struggle with this experience. However, it also gave me more resolve and strength to make sure that we did everything we could possibly do to help her with this transition and to find the most appropriate care for her. I also think that this experience helped me realize the most important thing was that she be in an environment where she would be content and find peace.

When we find the right facility for our loved one, it can be the beginning of healing for the entire family. What I learned by going to seminars, reading material, and talking with caregivers, was that it can be very healthy for the family members when someone else takes on the role of primary caregiver. There are many reasons for this. In my personal experience, my mother seems to be more comfortable and more compliant with her caregivers than she was with my sister and me.

People who work with dementia will always say that one never wins an argument with a person who has dementia. This makes a difficult dynamic when we are living with and caring for a family member. For example, in my situation, my mother was the matriarch of our family, so it was very difficult for my sister and me to attempt to have her do something that she insisted she did not want to do. In my old family dynamic, mom was the boss and my sister and I were very uncomfortable "making" mom do something against her will!

Furthermore, people with dementia have difficulty and fear surrounding things that we take for granted, such as basic functions of daily life. For example, toileting and hygiene create a tremendous amount of fear in someone who has dementia, and it is often helpful when the family members are not the ones responsible for this kind of care.

One might think that mom or dad would be willing to let us help them shower or brush their teeth, but at least in my experience, my mother is much more comfortable with her CNAs who provide this care than she ever was with me. When we did have my mother in the home, she seemed more comfortable letting the home-health aide help with basic care than one of the family. Having a health professional trained in dementia care helping our loved one allows the family to be the family. It gives us more freedom to foster connections that help bring comfort and peace to the one we love.

We were fortunate to find an amazing facility for my mother. The Alzheimer's Resource Center of Connecticut has a culture of healing and respect for all life. The entire staff is not only trained in dementia care, but also is aware of and responsive to the individual needs of each resident. I believe that my mother's spirit has been healed by living in this environment. While I love this facility and staff, it continues to be difficult for me to leave my mother after a visit. Once when she was new to the facility, she asked, "Can I come sleep at your house?" That was painful for me to hear, and it was more painful when I once again had to say, "This is where you live, Mom." After more than two years, it is still hard for me to leave my mother, but only because I miss her. Because she lives at the Center, our family is able to feel comfortable and secure in the awareness that she receives the best care possible, is loved by the staff, and is connected to her community and fellow residents. She is content and has found peace.

Primary caregiver

If we do decide to be the primary caregiver for our loved one, we need to also take care of ourselves. Being a caregiver to our loved one is a choice that many of us make, and with this choice comes a lot of stress. Being responsible for the health and welfare of someone with dementia is a 24-hour, 7-day-a-week job. It involves making sure that our loved one has the appropriate medical care, maintains a regimented schedule for medication, ensuring their safety, hygiene, proper nutrition, providing meaningful interaction and activity, detecting shifts in decline, etc. Therefore it is imperative that we have a support system in place to help us when there is a crisis and also on an ongoing, daily basis, so that we are able to stay rested and healthy. A support system can consist of family, friends, a support group, or a church family. It is important for the care giver to be able and willing to ask for help and to let their support system know what they need.

Care plan

Being the primary caregiver to a loved one can be very stressful and depleting in a variety of ways, financially, spiritually, physically, and emotionally. One thing that we can do to help reduce our stress is to have a care plan for our loved one and to ask our support system to help us carry out that plan. Having a conference call every three months to our support people gives us a chance to check in and see how everything is going. That can be very helpful and gets more people involved in the care of our loved one. It helps caregivers feel they are supported and keeps everyone focused and reminded of the need for more than one person's involvement and responsibility for our loved one's care.

A care plan consists of identifying as many aspects of care as possible. When putting together a care plan, consider the following:

1- **Emergency plan**. An emergency plan would include identifying a hospital of preference, if there is one, a list of medications that are clearly marked and accessible if 911 needs to be called, having a medical alert bracelet on our loved one, a list of physicians, family phone numbers posted by the phone, a device that will call 911 if we are not able to reach a phone, a neighbor who has a key to our house, a person identified to look after a pet. Also indicate whether or not your loved one wants CPR or has completed advanced directives paperwork.

2- **Medical Records**. These will include diagnoses, prescriptions, supplements, and medical history. They can also include general observations that may be helpful for future care and an overview of general care given at home.

3- **Medical Care**. A description of medical care such as full, partial or assisted care, a list of home health aides and their contact info, and day programs if our loved one is attending any. It is also important to have a medical power of attorney in place.

4- **Nutrition and diet**. Part of staying healthy is maintaining a balanced diet that includes fresh fruits and vegetables and the proper amount of fluids. If our loved one is gaining or losing weight due to activity level or as a side effect from a medication, their diet needs to be adjusted.

5- **Activities**. Keeping a list of possible activities can help us when we are overstressed and need to find something for our loved one to do, such as folding laundry, coloring, etc. There are also a variety of alternative therapies and activities that can have a positive impact on our loved one such as Chi Gong, Yoga, Reiki (which is a form of energy work), music, aroma, massage and pet therapy. Keeping a log of their activities helps us keep track of whether or not our loved one is being adequately engaged in life. If our loved one likes to be physically active, we might be able to hire someone to come and walk with them during the day and in the evening to help them expend some of their energy. Physical activity can have a very positive effect on the emotional wellbeing of our loved one. There is evidence that supports the fact that physical exercise can relieve the symptoms of depression and anxiety.

6- **Evaluation and Assessment.** Having a social worker or person trained in dementia care come in periodically to do a depression assessment on our loved one can also help us know if our care plan needs to be adjusted. It is also helpful to have our loved one's physician review our care plan on a regular basis. A care plan can highlight needs, give an opportunity for increased involvement from our support system, and bring us peace of mind.

HEALING FOR EVERYONE

Healing

"A Bird does not sing because it has an answer. It sings because it has a song." -Chinese proverb

Beyond Illness

The Greek word for healing means "to restore." Usually, when we think of restoring something, we think of making it like it used to be. We restore old houses and cars and things that are broken by fixing them. However, when our understanding of healing includes "fixing," it can impede our ability to believe in the possibility of healing the life of someone who has Alzheimer's and dementia. It is possible to heal the life of someone who has dementia. However, in order for this to happen, we must remember that all life needs to be nurtured and loved, not fixed. It does not mean that their cognitive abilities are restored, but that their sense of peace and connection are being nurtured. For a person with dementia, healing occurs when their life and spirit are celebrated and nurtured.

Disease versus illness

In his book, *The Birth of Christianity*, John Dominic Crossan quotes Leon Eisenberg from *Disease and Illnesses*, citing:

> *Illnesses are experiences of disvalued changes in states of being and in social function; diseases, in the scientific paradigm of modern medicine, are abnormalities in the structure and function of bodily organs and systems. We cure diseases, but we heal illnesses.*

We can heal the illness of dementia by maintaining our awareness that the beauty of life exists regardless of one's ability.

Our world, culture, and society all disvalue states of being by saying that our lives must fit in to a predetermined and preapproved box. It disvalues some lives while valuing others. Gender, socioeconomic class, education, age, and ethnicity are all part of the value judgments given to us by society. We label people based on the circumstances of their lives and then make judgments about the quality of those lives. Often when people are labeled with a disease, they lose the other facets of their lives and, in a sense, become one-dimensional to those around them. When my mother was diagnosed with dementia, I hesitated to tell anyone, because I was trying to protect her from "becoming" her disease. I tried to protect her from having a value judgment placed on her life because of her disease. She already had a disease; she did not need an illness on top of it!

When we judge another person or disvalue his or her life, we bring illness to that person. Yet we all have the capacity to heal those around us and, ultimately, our world when we know that a life has value and worth just because it "is." We can heal our life and heal the world by changing the experiences of those around us, by embracing the life that is before us, and by honoring the inherent value that we have all been given.

Healing energy

Healing energy is a continual life-sustaining process that is present in every moment. It moves in us and through us regardless of our abilities. Even though the universe moves all things toward balance and wholeness, this healing energy can get blocked by how we live with one another. Our participation in healing is based on whether we chose to block or facilitate the healing process. We facilitate healing by being a vessel through which healing energy can move and be directed. For this to happen, we need to believe in this possibility and believing in this possibility, for some of us, requires a shift in awareness. The more people who shift their awareness, the greater the possibility becomes.

Each person has an effect on the whole of life. A small change at one place in a complex system can have a large effect elsewhere.

The hundredth monkey

The Hundredth Monkey by Ken Keys JR. reports that in 1952, on the island of Koshima, scientists provided monkeys with sweet potatoes dropped in the sand. The monkeys liked the taste of the raw sweet potatoes, but they found the dirt unpleasant. An 18 month-old female named Imo found she could solve the problem by washing the potatoes in a nearby stream. She taught this trick to her mother. Her playmates also learned this new way, and they taught their mothers too. This cultural innovation was gradually picked up by various monkeys as the scientists watched and took notes. Between 1952 and 1958, all the young monkeys learned to wash the sandy sweet potatoes to make them more palatable. Only the adults who imitated their young learned this social improvement. Then, in the autumn of 1958, a certain number of monkeys were all washing the sweet potatoes and by evening almost all the monkeys were washing their sweet potatoes. They are suggesting that there were 99 monkeys washing the potatoes, but when the 100th monkey joined in, there was a shift. The added energy of the hundredth monkey somehow created an ideological shift or "tipping point."

Here's the biggest surprise. The habit of washing sweet potatoes then jumped over the sea. Colonies of monkeys on other islands and the mainland troop of monkeys at Takasakiyama all began washing their sweet potatoes. Thus, when a certain critical number achieves awareness, this new awareness may be communicated from mind to mind. There is a point at which if only one person tunes in to a new awareness, an energy field is strengthened, so this awareness is picked up by everyone.

The possibility of healing

"Awake my soul to the rhythm of our hearts, to the song of our love." Linn Possell

Beyond limits

What we find in our life is contingent upon where, and for what, we are looking. What and where we look comes from our belief about what we will find. If we look for limitations, believing not in infinite possibilities, but in limited possibilities, that is what we will find. If, however, we put no limitations on our search, then we will be open to the infinite possibilities that exist. One possibility that exists is the possibility of healing.

What do you believe about dementia? For what are you looking when you look at your mother, father, spouse, or sibling who has dementia? What is your focus when you look at your loved one? Are you open to the possibilities of healing and, if so, do you remain open to how these possibilities might present themselves?

Life is Limitless

When we look for possibilities, it is important to believe and trust that possibilities exist, because believing in limitations can hinder healing. Allow yourself to be committed to healing; knowing that every experience will be unique and recognizing that distractions might make it difficult to remain open. One potential distraction that we have is seeing our loved one as limited. As adults we believe in limitations. We believe that our world is limited, our lives are limited, time is limited, etc. We believe in the limitations taught to us by our culture and our world. Religion can limit us, our schools limit us, our abilities, our ethnicity, gender and age can limit us if we believe in the doctrine of limitations. But we do not have to experience life as limited.

Life is limitless. Therefore we can live a life that is limitless. What we give power to in our lives dictates our experience. The way that this happens is not by trying to overcome a limitation, but by refusing to see it as a limitation at all. When we think about overcoming a limitation, we give it power because we recognize the limitation as true. When we believe in the limitations of ourselves and of others, we live lives that are restricted, because we modify who we are. When that happens we miss out on the beauty of life and the beauty of the lives around us. Life is amazing and yet we might be missing it.

The only power that really exists is the power of love. Love goes beyond limits and connects with life as it is. Therefore, we can live a life without limits when we connect with the power of love. The power of love does not recognize barriers, limitations, abilities, or impairments. The power of love recognizes life.

Beyond ego

Ego is our attachment to and definition of "self." For many of us, our ego is defined by our actions and our power or lack of power to take action. For example, if my ego is defined by my ability to affect change in a situation at work or home, I will feel positive or negative about my "self" and who I am, depending on my success in creating that change. This is so because ego is our individual identity and our culture tells us that our identity is contingent upon what we do. Our ego can become a distraction and a stumbling block to the healing process, because when our sense of self is connected to an outcome, often times we shift our focus to the outcome rather than the process. When our intent is to facilitate healing, it is necessary for us to set our ego or sense of identity aside, and focus on the life-affirming energy that already exists in the world. When we free ourselves from ego, we are more open and able to connect with the energy of those that we love and the universal energy that creates healing.

Healing energy is limitless and affects everyone involved

How can we help the healing process?

Remember that healing is an interactive exchange of energy and requires that we honor the sacred in all of life.

1-To be aids in the process of healing, we must *form a connection* by entering in to the energetic space of the one who needs the healing. This means either meeting the person where they are literally or figuratively. We can connect energetically with another person by sending energy. 2-Healing energy needs *intent and focus* and can be shared with someone wherever they happen to be. 3-Healing also requires that we let ourselves be *vulnerable* to the situation and humble in the presence of the person with whom we are connecting. 4-Our response to one another changes how we interact and our *emotional response* to our loved one can affect their experience of life. When we try and protect ourselves, we build walls that are tough to penetrate. 5-To be a facilitator of healing, it is essential to be *without walls.* If we feel grief, anger, frustration, or any emotion that might get in the way of our capacity to be fully present, we need to try and release this emotion for at least the time that we are in their presence. 6-To be facilitators of healing, we also must *be open to the reality of the present moment* and not be distracted by the past or the future. So many times in our life we are busy preparing for the future that we fail to see what is going on in the present moment and we may also fail to see one another.

Therefore, we cannot be distracted by thoughts about the disease, what we need to do later in the day, or what happened in our lives before we came to see our loved one. 7-Healing is an exchange of energy. It is not something that we do *for* someone. When we are facilitating energy work, it is important to remember that the outcome is more dependent on the exchange of energy between "Spirit," God, or whatever name you give to the energy that calls life into being, and person undergoing the healing process. The facilitator is less important in this sacred energy exchange.

Freedom to be

The staff that cares for my mother gives her the freedom "to be." They understand that she is an individual and has unique manifestations of her disease. It often seems to me that when people are diagnosed with dementia and Alzheimer's, they are put in to a box and treated as if they are all alike. But that is not the case with someone who has dementia or Alzheimer's. Just as it is not the case with any life. We are all unique and deserve to be treated and loved as our own person.

The freedom to be is another form of healing and is an immeasurable gift that we can give to one another. We can give the freedom to be to those around us when we honor one another and believe that ALL life is sacred. In Hinduism, *Namaste* means, "I honor the sacred in you." It does not mean some aspects of you are sacred and other aspects are not. Namaste means that life's essence is sacred. I think that in the West we see people more as having parts that make up the whole person. We tend to say things like, "I love you unconditionally," which really means that "there are parts of you I have to overlook, so that I can love you." Thinking that a person is the sum of their parts leads to our understanding of unconditional love, rather than Namaste. "Loving freely" or loving "just because" is more closely related to Namaste. In the same way, honoring the sacred in one another means that life is sacred just because it *is*, and when we are able to embody that belief about life, we will be able to give others the freedom to be. The freedom to be not only frees a person from judgment and expectations, but also is a blessing for everyone involved.

Love

Healing, therefore, is a possibility that exists for all life, regardless of circumstance or situation. It requires openness, love, and the understanding that the essence of life is love.

Because the essence of life is love, we live this out when we focus our attention and energy on love. Life is not the finite pieces of our individual lives that create the boxes in which we place one another. Life is a creative process that is the ever unfolding energy of love. When we make a conscious choice to live in and be a part of this energy, then we allow ourselves and those around us the opportunity to live freely, without the labels and expectations that restrict our ability to tap into our energy of love. The possibilities of a new life for ourselves and for the people with whom we interact is a matter of choice.

WISDOM

Heart wisdom

"The spirit of life never dies. It is the infinite gateway to mysteries within mysteries." The Tao Te Ching

Beyond what is visible

Seeing beyond circumstances and connecting to the spirit is the way that we facilitate healing. To do this, we must go beyond perceptions and physical markers. The brain sees what is physical and can be distracted by what it sees. Therefore healing begins when we follow something more than the intellect and perceptions of the brain. Healing begins when we follow the wisdom of the heart.

Research shows that at least half the cells of the heart are neural cells like those found in the brain, and that the heart has its own intelligence. However, our heart knowledge involves a different kind of intelligence than we have become accustomed to using on a daily basis. It is possible to shift our intelligence and to utilize both the brain and the heart. The knowledge that resides in the heart is our awareness of our universal oneness, and this intelligence leads us toward wholeness and balance.

We are not used to listening to and living from the wisdom of our heart, and so the heart's intelligence can be blocked by the chatter in our brain. This happens by the tapes in our head that tell us the same story over and over again and often leads us into suffering. But if we are intentional and aware of the knowledge of our heart, and if we stay connected to that intelligence, the heart can create new awareness and new possibilities for life.

The heart's intelligence is not based in the time and space continuum as is the intellect in our head. The wisdom of the heart comes from imagination rather than cognitive intellect. Thus it is only limited by our capacity to imagine new possibilities of connection. This intelligence is also the intelligence of love. And because love is the energetic frequency that calls life into being, it is the heart that will help us when our loved one has Alzheimer's and dementia.

Energy connects with like energy

Love is the energy that nurtures and sustains life and it only synchronizes with the same energy. When we are in the presence of a person who has dementia, we can be assured that an intelligence exists of which they are still capable and with which we can connect. Deepak Chopra has stated that "We see what we vibrate to." If our vibrations are vibrations of love, that is what we will experience. If our energy is the energy of anger or frustration, then that will be our experience. To be able to see beyond the information brought into and processed by the brain, we must move into the intelligence of the heart. This is where our healing takes place.

I have no idea if my mother knows that I am her daughter or not, but I do know that she recognizes the energy that people bring when they interact with her. A cousin of mine asked me if my mother would recognize her if she were to visit. I said that I believed that my mother would recognize her energy. My mother responds to the energy of love and connectedness whomever it comes from. Energy connects with like energy and because of the facility where my mother lives and the staff who work with her, my mother is constantly surrounded by loving energy. To me, this is a great gift that allows me to trust that she is content with her life. We can still be a significant source of connection and joy for our loved one, even if we are new to them every time we visit. They respond to our energy, our smile, our touch. Being connected is a significant piece in the healing process, so it is important to try and convey to our loved one that they are significant enough for us to connect with them. Our interactions and connectedness will have a significant impact on their experience of life.

The memory of energy

People with dementia might not remember our visit or our presence cognitively, but they will remember it on an energetic level. Some scientists think that memories of experiences are stored in our cells. These memories are stored by the same chemical process that happens in the brain for cognitive memory. There are many reports of people with transplanted organs reacting to experiences and having personality traits of the donor, which demonstrates that our cells do hold a memory whether we are aware of this or not. We cannot know for sure what our loved one is experiencing, but if we accept the possibility that they are affected by their environment and can connect with those around them, we might see how important our contact is to their experience of life and ours too.

It has been demonstrated that in very young children, the primary caregiver's emotional state determines the child's state, and therefore the child's development in general. I believe that this is also true for people with cognitive changes.

Knowing

I see my mother using the intelligence of her heart. She is fully engaged in and aware of her life. Her intelligence comes from her heart and is responsive to the energy coming from those around her. I have watched members of other families speak to her and embrace her, and I have seen how she responds to their interaction without "knowing" them.

I live in Florida and my mother lives in Connecticut. I go up to see her every chance I get, but that still is only every other month. Even though I only see my mother every other month, she continues to be connected to me. When I first enter her living space, I stand or sit where she can see me. I watch as she looks at me, and I know it will take about ten minutes before she comes over to me. She then stands in front of me and begins to smile. I do not know what she is "thinking," but I do know that she is "knowing" that I am someone who loves and adores her, and someone to whom she remains connected. I believe that she is using the intelligence of her heart.

The last time that I saw my mother, about two weeks ago, she recognized me within seconds. This amazed me, because she had not seen me for two-and-a-half months, but after about thirty seconds of looking at me, her face lit up in a great smile. I am always a little worried that she will not recognize me when I first arrive. I have to take a moment to remind myself that the intent of my visit is to bring positive, healing energy to her and to infuse this energy with her environment.

What was also great about my last visit to see my mother was that when I entered the unit where she lives, she was sitting at the lunch table holding her roommate's daughter's hand. One of the things that is wonderful about the facility where my mother lives is the philosophy built around their saying, "we live it with you." This philosophy is embraced by many family members as well, and we interact with all of the residents, not just our loved one.

How can we shift into positive energy?

"Our task must be to widen our circle of compassion, to embrace all living creatures and the whole of nature in its beauty." Albert Einstein

Centering

When we enter into any situation, it is always beneficial to find our own "center," so that we can be fully present. Finding our center means to connect with and focus on our source. When we focus on our emotion or on how we feel about a situation or if we have a desired goal or objective in mind, we are not free to be fully present to allow the moment of living to happen. Centering our self in our source, or God, keeps us focused on the beauty of life. Goals and objectives are things that we manipulate into being. Being fully present allows life to unfold in its own way.

Finding our center grounds us, helps us calm our emotions, and gives us strength with any situation in our lives. This can be especially helpful before we visit with a person who has dementia. When we become cognizant about our intentions about who we are and what kind of energy we want to bring to a situation, it has a way of centering us and reminding us of the importance of our energy. This will have a positive effect on everyone involved.

Attachment to an outcome

An intention for a desired outcome will not necessarily have a positive effect. When we are attached to a specific outcome, it is difficult to be fully present because we focus on the outcome rather than the interaction. If I am trying to get another person to understand my point of view or if I want that person to respond in a certain way, my focus will be on trying to persuade or manipulate them, so that I can accomplish my goal. This also prevents us from being fully present.

Being present

Being fully present enables us to be fully engaged and connected with one another. Trying to change someone is a form of manipulation that happens when we try to get a person to do, say, or experience something, rather than allowing life to unfold .When we allow life to unfold without being restricted by ideas of what we want or think should happen, we are more able to connect with one another. When we spend time with our loved one in this way, we will become more aware of the beauty of their life.

CONNECTING WITH THE SPIRIT

Prayer

"When you pray, move your feet." African proverb

Prayer is another way of shifting into healing energy. We have a variety of ways in which we think about prayer, and the meaning of prayer is different for different people. I believe that the way we think about prayer has major implications for our lives and for the lives of those around us. Why we pray, what we focus on when we pray, and what we believe can happen when we pray, all have significant implications for our lives.

I believe that some popular ideas and beliefs about prayer can lead to destructive consequences. For instance, we must remember that prayer is not isolated and does impact those around us and other forms of life. If we pray to win a war, we must remember that death for other people is necessary for that prayer to be realized. A prayer that does not help balance all of life is one in which we ask a power with the ability and willingness to be subjective and selective, to grant our prayers at the cost of others.

Sometimes we pray because we think that we can coax satisfaction out of the universe or from God. Many people assume that we can appease or flatter God by using the right words and that when we use the correct words, God will listen to and grant our petition. The function of prayer is to open ourselves up to God's interactions with us. Prayer can be a time for focusing on our relationships and overcoming the obstacles we face. Prayer can be used to learn to live in the presence of love. Prayer can help us absorb the presence of love within our own lives. Prayer affects our whole being; it affects those around us; it affects the whole world. Therefore we pray for healing not to ensure recovery, but to align ourselves with the presence of love and wholeness that is already at work in the universe. What do you pray for when you pray for your loved one with dementia?

Becoming our prayer

Prayer is a way that we can change on an energetic level, that enables us to bring an intention into our being, which becomes part of who we are. Prayer becomes reality when we become our prayer. Becoming our prayer means that we breathe life in to the prayer, and we do this by *becoming* peace, *becoming* a healing presence, *embodying* compassion etc. Prayer is about how we live our lives. I tell people that I know what it is they pray for, when I see what they live. Prayer is more than taking a moment to talk to God or the universe. Our life is our prayer.

When I pray for my mother, I pray for her to experience peace and contentment. My prayer begins when I focus on how peace and contentment feels within me, then I bring to mind an image of my mother in all aspects of her life where she lives. I pray for her to have peace as she sleeps, as she is cared for by her CNAs. I pray for her to experience peace while she engages in the activities where she lives and as she connects with her community.

Soren Kierkegaard said, "Prayer does not change God, but changes him who prays." Prayer is more than trying to get the universe or God to adjust to our wishes. Rather, it is about us trying to embody our prayer. For example, if we pray for peace and bring the energy of peace into our body, mind, and spirit, then we will become peace and bring peace to the world. This is how our prayers will be realized, and this is how our life becomes our prayer.

Be the change

"Be the change you wish to see in the world." Ghandi.

"The world will not change until we change." Marianne Williamson

"We cannot solve the problems of the world from the level of thinking we were at when we created them." Einstein

"If you do not change direction, you may end up where you are heading." Lao Tsu

These teachers from different places around the world, from different cultures, and from different times, all agree that in order for things to change around us, we must change. Prayer helps us to do just that, because prayer changes who we are.

Prayer is about life, change, imagination, and action. Prayer is an experience and therefore, is interactive, transformative, and ongoing. What do we hear when we hear our teachers talk about prayer? Do we hear that prayer requires using the appropriate words or about making a good argument in order to persuade God to act in some way? I do not hear anything like that when I listen to the teachings of Jesus, Buddha, or Lao Tzu, or even from our more contemporary teachers quoted above. When I listen to the teachings of prayer, I hear that it is an exchange of energy between God and ourselves, between us and creation and between individuals. Prayer is an exchange of energy and involves not praying for a specific outcome, but for a new possibility, whatever that may be. For those who believe in a Higher Power, we know it is sometimes difficult to understand what is "best" in life. We also trust that this life is not the only life that we have.

Prayer is transformative because it involves change. Prayer changes us when we open ourselves to seeing something differently. We are changed when we see or imagine the possibility that something could be different. However, this change does not happen when we look at something and think that *it needs* to change. Thinking that something needs to change is judging a person or circumstance. Rather, change happens when we imagine a different, more life-affirming possibility, not when we think someone or something should change because we have judged or measured it to be wrong or undesirable.

It has been demonstrated that prayer has an effect on us. There are specific areas of the brain that light up on a Positron Emission Tomogrophy (PET) scan when we pray. Experiments have shown that when one person prayed for another who was in a separate room and completely unaware that they were the focus of the prayer, both subjects' brains lit up at exactly the same time: when the prayer began.

Prayer changes both the person praying and the person for whom the prayer is given. Three years ago I embarked on a vision quest and ran a 100-mile race in Africa. As I trained and told people about my race, they asked me why I was running. My answer was, "Because I can." I thought that was a good enough answer and reason for doing something. While I was training, I thought to myself, "How great is it that I am able to do something just because I can." And then I began to think about my 10-year-old niece who had Juvenile Rheumatoid Arthritis (JRA).

JRA is a very painful, sometimes crippling disease and my niece, Lexi, had a severe case. It was so severe, she had to travel twice a month to a hospital four hours each way, for eight hours of infusion therapy. No one could really say what the side effects of this treatment would be, but it was the only thing that seemed to work for her. She struggled to go to school and could no longer engage in the activities she loved.

It occurred to me that Lexi was not able to do something "just because she could," and so I turned my run into a race for her and to raise awareness for JRA. The other thing that I did was ask my congregation to send her positive energy I asked them to tell people about Lexi and JRA and asked that before they set out to do something "just because they can," whether that was to take a walk, ride a bike, play golf, etc. that they imagine a day that my niece would be able to do so as well. We focused our positive energy for a year while I trained for my race, and many people in my congregation continue to send Lexi positive energy. We imagined a different life for my niece, we imagined a new possibility for her, and three years later, Lexi is off all her medications and able to do things "just because she can." While she is doing much better, she is still unable to do all of the activities that interest her, but her life has changed, and those of us who imagined a different possibility for Lexi have also been changed.

What is your prayer for your loved one with dementia? Can you imagine a different reality for his or her life? How do you need to change for that to happen?

Creating space for connection to take place

"At the heart of each of us, whatever our imperfections, there exists a silent pulse of perfect rhythm, which is absolutely individual and unique, and yet which connects us to everything else."
George Leonard

An electromagnetic field radiates from our heart. This energy field encompasses our entire body and can extend out for up to fifteen feet. When we are in close proximity to another person, we can often feel their energy, because the energetic field is strongest within three feet from the heart. This energetic field provides the power and gives us the capability of connecting with another living being. Whether we use this power and capability is up to us. The energetic field of the heart is not limited by a decrease in our cognitive ability. Therefore, we can have a meaningful connection with our loved one that leads us both toward wholeness and balance.

Some of the emotions we feel when a loved one has dementia include sadness, frustration, guilt, and anger. These emotions come from our grief over the losses that come from this disease. However, when we fuel the energy of these emotions, we create distance between family members and also with the one who has the disease. When we look at loss and place a measurement on it, we create separation. Placing a measurement on someone puts a barrier between us and prevents connection. If our intention is to connect, there must be an open space between us for the connection to take place. We must open the door for that possibility to enter.

We experience life differently

People with dementia might experience life in new ways. What once was interesting may not hold much or any interest to them now. Our idea of how someone usually experiences life may not correspond with how they experience life. Since my mother used to be a very busy person, always involved in activities like swimming, gardening, or reading, etc., I thought when she moved into a facility for people with dementia, that she still needed to be involved in a lot of activities. I used to call and question the activities coordinator to make sure that mom was doing "enough" to stay happy and engaged. What I have come to realize is that my mother's need to be active and involved is not the same as before. I used to think that when I visited my mother, I needed to always be doing something with her, but this has changed as well. I now know and am comfortable with the fact that sitting and holding her hand is what she wants me to do, even if it is for hours at a time. She has demonstrated that this interaction is enough and is what is best for her. When we visit our loved one, we may need to adjust our perception and expectation of the visit. This will help release both parties from expectations of what "should" happen during our time together.

One time while visiting my mother, I observed an interaction between a son and father. The son had brought along some of the father's favorite candy and a book that he used to love. The father, however, was not very responsive and kept falling asleep, which made the son very anxious. This was difficult to watch, because I knew that the son really wanted to have a meaningful time with his father. The father, however, seemed very comfortable and peaceful as he slept in his chair. Of course when we visit our loved one, we want them to know that we have come that we care about and love them. We also want our visit to be meaningful and to feel connected to them. However, there comes a time with this disease, when we need to change our perception of what we mean by the word "meaningful."

Connection

I now understand that connection comes in many forms, and whether we perceive our loved one as knowing that we are visiting or not, they do have a level of awareness that enables them to connect with us. They recognize our presence on an energetic level. They feel our presence with the awareness of the heart. If we find our loved one sleeping when we come to visit, we can notice whether they are comfortable, we can sit with them and pray, we can massage their hands or their feet, or we can speak to them as if they were awake. I find myself doing this more often with my mother now that she her disease has progressed to a more advanced stage. Connecting with the spirit does not depend on wakefulness, only openness.

Spirit

"Be aware of that which is right in front of you; then you will be able to grasp what is out of your sight. For there is nothing hidden that will not be known." The Gospel of Thomas

The words spirit and love are interchangeable. Love is eternal and cannot be hindered by what is merely physical. Love and spirit are what is real and eternal in this world. In Judaism, the word "Ruach" means wind or spirit. It is said that this divine breath moved across the creation and into it breathed life. Our spirit is the essence of our being; it breathes life into our physical experience. We nourish our spirit by the way we live our lives. What we do, how we interact with other people, the thoughts we have, the experiences of our lives, all affect the spirit. Spirit can be touched when we are aware of the sacredness of every life and of each moment.

Sometimes we may feel unconnected or unaffected by spirit. But this happens when we focus on what we believe to be reality that exists within the normal realm of life. In the Celtic tradition, it is believed that there are "thin places" where the normal and the divine meet. In a "thin place" we are able to connect with the divine. Two examples of physical thin places are: where water and land meet at the shore and in the twilight hour where day and night meet. If we believe that the divine is present in our daily lives, then wherever we experience this feeling and awareness of the sacred is a thin place. Whenever we are able to connect with another person, we are in a thin place. To do this, it is necessary for us to believe in the possibility of the sacred in one another.

Beyond separation

There is a theory that claims that we are all only six degrees of separation apart from anyone else in the world. We welcome this theory because we live in an elaborate system of separation, which we have accepted as true. Now we feel good to think we are only six steps away from all other people. Why does this notion make us feel so good? Because we believe in separation when in fact there is no separation. Life is ultimately connected at all times. Whatever separation we feel, whatever barriers we perceive, they are made up out of our own creations. Reality lies not in what we have created, but in what God has created. Life and connectedness are the only reality, and we will find this to be true when we look for ways in which life is connected. If we can imagine going beyond what society tells us are the impairments that come with dementia, we will discover new possibilities for life. We will find connectedness and joy. It is possible to have a rich and wonderful relationship with people who have dementia.

Characteristics, abilities, and appearances are all outside layers of an individual. What we find under these layers is the spirit. The spiritual essence of a person is, essentially fundamentally, the essence of life. It connects us to all of life. The spirit is eternal, and when our loved one has dementia, we can use this as an opportunity to explore how to connect with one another through the spirit.

Looking for the Spirit

"We are not human beings having a spiritual experience. We are spiritual beings having a human experience." Telliard de Chardin

It seems as if we venture out on a spiritual path when we seek something more than what we are experiencing in our daily lives. What we usually are looking for is a feeling or experience of fulfillment that comes from knowing about or connecting to what we have come to define as God. A spiritual path for growth and awareness leads to a place of peace. Spiritual growth can lead us to a greater awareness of our spirit and our soul. Spirit is the energy that exists in life and transcends all things. Spirit is what we call the universal life force, the numinous, God. It is at the same time in all things and beyond all things. It is what connects all of life. Spirit exists in the very core of our being, as well as in the star dust of the galaxies, and in the stem of a flower. It draws rivers to the ocean and makes up the drops of water. Spirit is in all life and is eternal.

Spiritual paths

Spiritual paths are important to our lives and to the way we live, because they help us focus on more than ourselves. They help us go beyond ego and become fully present in each moment of our lives. Spirituality is our experience of something other than the "self" of ego. A spiritual path helps us focus and relate to this presence and enables us to form our understanding of life. When Telliard De Chardin writes that "We are spiritual beings having a human experience," this statement can help us look at one another differently; it reminds us that life is more than what we generally perceive. When someone has dementia, at some point he or she may not be able to fully engage in this "human experience," but they still remain spiritual beings.

Our spiritual path is the lens through which we see, understand, and relate to the experience of something greater than ourselves, which many of us call God. The wisdom teachers, around which many religions have formed, and that many of us follow, all show us that life is meant to be lived in union and compassion with one another and with God. Therefore we are asked to live life by being aware of other life around us and to consider the implications of our actions.

Soul

Our soul is the part of our essence that is unique and finds expression in the world. Soul is very personal and yet exists beyond our physical bodies. Therefore, soul goes beyond ego, because our ego is attached to the material world. The ego is driven by our belief in cultural norms and the framing of religions that give us the measurements that shape our belief about who and how we are in the world. Soul is not contingent upon these things. Soul is the intuitive "knowing" we have when we cannot identify where our knowledge originated. We have touched our soul when we feel grounded and certain of our path. Soul exists in the heart and is the core of our being, which can be expressed in our gifts and abilities, our characteristics and personality, but it goes beyond these as well.

A person with dementia expresses themselves differently in the world. However, their souls continue to find expression; they are capable of experiencing peace, and they remain open to joy. When these individuals are treated as if their souls can no longer be expressed and others believe they have lost their ability to connect with spirit, their life begins to fade. The disease does not rob a person with dementia of their life, their soul and their spirit. What robs them is when we fail to give them the grace to find new expression and when we stop looking for new ways to help them connect with life. The essence of life continues to move toward growth and awareness. What is eternal is the spirit and the soul. Therefore, when someone has dementia, their spirit and soul continue to be. We can facilitate this growth and awareness when we set aside our preconceived ideas about Alzheimer's and dementia, and give them the grace to find new expression, continue to stay connected, and recognize and celebrate their... *Beautiful Spirit.*

May the sun bring you energy by day, may the moon softly restore you by night, may the rain wash away your worries, may the breeze blow new strength into your being. May you walk gently through the world and know its beauty all the days of your life.

Apache blessing

EPILOGUE

Four weeks ago I received a call from the facility where my mother lived. I remember thinking that this time the message did not begin with, "everything is ok". I was being called because there was a significant change in my mother's condition. The change was that my mom was not eating or drinking. Six months ago my mother lost the ability to feed herself because she could not complete the entire sequence of scooping food on to her spoon, bringing it to her mouth, taking the food in and swallowing. When we think about what we perceive as the simplest tasks, we often forget how detailed they really are.

I was told that sometimes people will refuse to eat at the end of life but this was not the case with my mother. She lost the ability to eat and drink. Mom would sip a spoonful of liquid or food into her mouth, she would swallow but could not get the food far enough back that the food would go down her throat. The change in my mother's condition was not a conscious choice. However, there were other choices that she continued to make even as she began her transition from this life to the next. And there were choices that we made as well as we began to prepare for her transition. One choice was to surround my mother with love, music and touch. We took her out in her wheelchair to the butterfly garden and walked for hours listening to her favorite classical guitar music on my iphone. We gave her foot and hand massages to prevent anxiety and bring comfort and had many conversations with her about our life and our love for her. We played a Triple Mantra protective sound current to help fill the room with peace and played her Carrie Newcomer's song, "The Gathering of Spirits". We made the choice to connect with my mother's spirit in every way we could.

Windows are moments of clarity that a person with dementia has at times. I have heard stories of people being able to speak to their loved ones at their time of death. I was hoping that when the time came my mother would be able to say something to us. Instead of spoken words, we were gifted with my mother taking long moments to look into each one of our eyes for the week of her transition. My mother intentionally looked into the eyes of each person who was there and we could all feel the depth her spirit as she seemed to be talking to and really connecting with us. She was speaking to us from the wisdom of her heart and making sure that she saw us and that we could also see her. My mother was making sure that we could see her spirit so that we would recognize it when we no longer could see her beautiful eyes looking at us, teaching us and loving us.

My mother did not make the choice to stop eating but she did make other choices. On the day that she died mom was doing pretty well and her slow decline left the staff thinking that it would be a few more days before she passed. I was sitting in her room with my sisters and talking with some of her caregivers who had become our sisters as well when I asked the question we had asked every day. "Will you all be working tomorrow?" Mom's caregivers were so amazing and she had such as strong connection with them that we wanted to make sure that they would be there to help her with her transition. I was disheartened to hear that the ones who she was closest to were all going to be off the next day. So I said to my mother, "Mom... Donna, Brittany, Janine, Doris, Lori and the rest will not be here tomorrow. If you want them to be with you and with us then you are going to need to hang in there for a couple more days. Or if you want them to be with you and us you can choose to go today." Within twenty minutes my mother made her final transition from this life.

My mother created a bond with each one of her family and caregivers during that final week of her human experience that, if we were looking, will continue to help guide us throughout our life and keep us connected to her spirit. For those of us that were looking, we are able to recognize the individual spark that is her soul as she continues to be present in this dimension and beyond. When I need help, I close my eyes and look into her beautiful green eyes again. This helps me touch the place in my heart where our souls meet and as our souls meet, I can again join her spirit in the flow of energy that is the eternal source of life.

Several years ago my mother faced one of her biggest challenges and embarked on one of her most important triumphs when she was diagnosed with dementia. Her triumph was the triumph of the spirit, because she continued to be who she was. She always taught us that it isn't what you do but who you are that matters. While she was affected physically she was unaffected spiritually. Her human experience changed but the essence of her being remained the same. It was a celebration of joy every time I was in her presence and this continued to be true while we all prepared for her to transition. One night one of her nurses came in, looked at my mother and said..."A class act right up until the end." Another commented that mom was going to be teaching us how to "get it right" even as she passed away. And that is what she did. My mother was and still is a beautiful spirit that touched many lives and taught me my most important lessons. She taught me that our spirit transcends everything, because it is the essence of life and that the bond of our spirit is as strong as it has ever been. Thank you mom, for teaching me my most valuable lesson.

RESOURCES

Alzheimer's Resource Center of CT. <u>Dining with Friends: An Innovative Approach to Dining for People with Dementia.</u> Arc-ct.org

Basting, Ann and David. <u>Forget Memory.</u> The Johns Hopkins University Press, 2009.

Beerman, Susan. <u>Eldercare 911 – The Caregiver's Complete Handbook for Making Decisions</u> . Prometheus Books, 2002.

Bell, Virginia. Troxel, David. <u>The Best Friends Approach.</u> Baltimore: Health Professions, 2002.

Cohen, Elizabeth. <u>The House on Beartown Road –A Memoir of Learning and Forgetting</u>. Random House, 2003.

Dunn, Hank. <u>Hard Choices for Loving People.</u> Lansdowne, VA: A and A Publishing, 2010.

Fiel, Naomi. <u>The Validation Breakthrough.</u> Health Professions, 2002

Fox, Judith. <u>I Still do.</u> Power House Books, 2009.

Genova, Lisa. <u>Still Alice.</u> New York, NY: Pocket Books, 2009.

Hoblitzelle, Olivia. <u>Ten Thousand Joys, Ten Thousand Sorrows.</u> NY: Tarcher, 2010.

Mace, Nancy. Peter, Rabins. <u>The 36 hour Day.</u> New York, Boston: Grand Central Publishing, 2001.

McCullough, Dennis. <u>MY MOTHER YOUR MOTHER Embracing "Slow Medicine," The Compassionate</u>

Approach To Caring For Your Aging Loved Ones. New York: Harper publishing, 2008.

McLay, Evelyn. Mom's Okay, She Just Forgets – A Handbook for Families. Prometheus Books, 2006.

Mex Glazner, Gerry. Editor. Sparkling Memories The Alzheimer's Poetry Project. Alzpoetry.com

Mitchell, Karyn. Reiki A Torch In Daylight, Spiritual Reiki . Oregon, IL: Mind Rivers Publishing, 2006.

Papa, Smith and Smith. Emotional Memory (article in Advance for Long Term Care Management Sept/Oct 2010)

Power, Al. MD. Dementia Beyond Drugs. Baltimore: Health Professions, 2010.

Radin, Lisa and Gary (edited by). What If It's Not Alzheimer's– A Caregivers Guide to Dementia. Prometheus Books, 2008.

Shapiro, Ed and Deb. BE THE CHANGE How meditation can transform you and the world. New York: Sterling publishing, 2009.

Whitehouse MD, Peter. The Myth of Alzheimer's Disease. St. Martins Press, 2008.

GLOSSARY

Affect – (noun) a set of observable manifestations of a subjectively experienced emotion.

Channel - a way, course, or direction of thought or action.

Cognitive - of, relating to, being, or involving conscious intellectual activity.

Compassion - a sympathetic consciousness of others' distress with desire to alleviate it.

Communal - of or relating to a community.

Communication - a unified body of individuals, a society at large.

Cope - to deal with and attempt to overcome problems and difficulties.

Cortisol - a glucocorticoid produced by the adrenal cortex, has anti-inflammatory and immunosuppressive properties, and whose levels in the blood may become elevated in response to physical or psychological stress.

Dualism - a doctrine that the universe is under the dominion of two opposing principles one of which is good and the other evil.

Early onset dementia – an uncommon form of dementia that strikes people younger than age 65.

Ego - the self especially as contrasted with another self or the world.

Empathy - the action of understanding, being aware of, being sensitive to, and vicariously experiencing the feelings, thoughts, and experience of another of either the past or present without having the feelings, thoughts, and experience fully communicated in an objectively explicit manner.

Energy - a usually positive spiritual force.

Essence - the most significant element, quality, or aspect of a thing or person.

Eternal - having infinite duration.

Healing - to make sound or whole.

Immune system - the bodily system that protects the body from foreign substances.

Judgment - the process of forming an opinion or evaluation by discerning and comparing.

Morality - a doctrine or system of moral conduct.

Peace - freedom from disquieting or oppressive thoughts or emotions.

Sacred - entitled to reverence and respect.

Soul - the immaterial essence, animating principle, or activating cause of an individual life.

Spirit - an animating or vital principle held to give life to physical organisms.

Stages of dementia

Stigma - a mark of shame or discredit.

Sympathy - an affinity, association, or relationship between persons or things wherein whatever affects one similarly affects the other.

Transfer - to convey from one person, place, or situation to another.

(Definitions adapted from Webster's Dictionary)

Alzheimer's and dementia information

Alzheimer's disease - a brain disease that impairs the brain's normal functioning. Deficits are represented by various symptoms and behavioral changes.

Dementia - a group of symptoms including; loss of memory, loss of judgment, loss of reason, loss of language, loss of time, loss of personality, overreacting to overwhelming situations.

Types of dementia disease, Lewy Body, Multi-Infarct (vascular), Frontotemporal (Picks), Parkinson's.

Related behaviors - Denial of problems, aggression, anxiety or agitation, confusion, repetition, suspicion, wandering, trouble with sleep, losing/hiding things, clinging behavior, inappropriate sexual behavior or comments.

Tips for Caregivers (Provided by Alzheimer's and Dementia Resource Center of Orlando www.ADRCcares,org).

Do...

Keep things as simple as possible.

Give instructions one step at a time.

Keep your loved one occupied with simple chores.

Remember they will follow you around and want to know where you are at all times.

Maintain a daily, structured routine.

Minimize distractions, noise and confusion.

Provide memory aids and cues when possible.

Be gentle – provide affection and support.

Maintain a sense of humor and acknowledge the small successes.

Get respite time away from your role as a caregiver.

Don't...

Expect answers to your questions to be accurate.

Get irritated when they ask the same question over and over.

Give them too much responsibility.

Expect then to properly identify people, places, or things.

Get upset, raise your voice or scold your loved one.

Take the person's behavior personally - it is a disease.

Argue with your loved one to try to rationalize with them.

(You will never win an argument with someone who has dementia.)

Expect...

To have normal feelings such as guilt, anger, sorrow, or helplessness.

Sleep disturbances.

Symptoms to worsen in the evening.

Behavior changes when there are major changes in daily life.

ABOUT THE AUTHOR

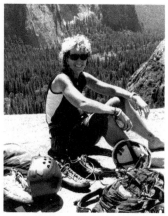

Rev Linn Possell is the consultant for Older Adult Ministry for the Florida Conference of the United Church of Christ in helping local churches better serve and engage the 60 - and - better population by providing training in congregational care, intergenerational programming, facilitating workshops in spiritual connectedness and offering resources to local clergy. She has been an ordained minister for ten years, is the founding pastor of Hope Unites UCC in Orlando FL, a Reiki Master, and leads workshops on communication and problem-solving for both the UCC and her local school districts. Linn has been counseling and providing support for families who have been affected by Alzheimer's and dementia for the past four years and manages a Facebook caregiver support group. Her mother was diagnosed with frontotemporal dementia in 2006.

ORDERING INFORMATION

To get additional copies of this book contact Rev. Linn Possell at revpossell@gmail.com or visit her web site at www.linnpossell.com

CPSIA information can be obtained
at www.ICGtesting.com
Printed in the USA
FFHW020924121118
49327817-53598FF